D0728469

Mayo Clinic on Managing Diabetes

Maria Collazo-Clavell, M.D.

Medical Editor in Chief

Mayo Clinic

Rochester, Minnesota

NEW HANOVER COUNTY
PUBLIC LIBRARY
201 CHESTNUT STREET
WILMINGTON, NC 28401

Mayo Clinic on Managing Diabetes provides reliable, practical, easy-to-understand information on controlling diabetes and preventing complications of the disease. Much of this information comes directly from the experience of endocrinologists and other health care professionals at Mayo Clinic. This book supplements the advice of your physician, whom you should consult for individual medical problems. *Mayo Clinic on Managing Diabetes* does not endorse any company or product. MAYO, MAYO CLINIC, MAYO CLINIC HEALTH INFORMATION and the Mayo triple-shield logo are marks of Mayo Foundation for Medical Education and Research.

Published by Mayo Clinic Health Information, Rochester, Minn. Distributed to the book trade by Kensington Publishing Corp., New York, N.Y. For bulk sales to employers, member groups and health-related companies, contact Mayo Clinic Health Management Resources, 200 First St. S.W., Rochester, MN 55905, or send e-mail to SpecialSalesMayoBooks@Mayo.edu.

Photo credits: Photos on Parts 1 and 3 © Stockbyte. Photos on Parts 2, 4, 5 and pages 60, 79, 94, 157, 195, 213 © Photodisc.

© 2006, Mayo Foundation for Medical Education and Research

All rights reserved. No part of this book may be reproduced or used in any form or by any means, electronic or mechanical, including photocopying and recording, or by any information storage and retrieval system, except for brief, attributed quotations, without permission in writing from the publisher. Address inquiries to Mayo Clinic Health Information, Permissions Department, 200 First St. S.W., Fifth Floor Centerplace Building, Rochester, MN 55905.

Library of Congress Catalog Card Number: 2005925743

ISBN-13: 978-1-893005-38-9
ISBN-10: 1-893005-38-0

Printed in the United States of America

Second Edition

1 2 3 4 5 6 7 8 9 10

About diabetes

More Americans than ever before have diabetes. The disease affects an estimated 21 million adults and children in the United States. And many people with diabetes don't have their disease under control. This is unfortunate because researchers continue to identify methods to better manage this common disease. Unlike years ago, today if you receive a diagnosis of diabetes, you have a good chance of living an active and healthy life — provided you work with your health care team to take the necessary steps to control your blood sugar.

Within these pages you'll find practical advice you can use to successfully manage your diabetes and reduce your risk of serious complications. If you're at risk of the disease, you'll learn about lifestyle changes that may keep you from developing diabetes. This book is based on the expertise of Mayo Clinic doctors and the advice they give day in and day out in caring for their patients.

About Mayo Clinic

Mayo Clinic evolved from the frontier practice of Dr. William Worrall Mayo and the partnership of his two sons, William J. and Charles H. Mayo, in the early 1900s. Pressed by the demands of their busy practice in Rochester, Minn., the Mayo brothers invited other physicians to join them, pioneering the private group practice of medicine. Today, with more than 2,000 physicians and scientists at its three major locations in Rochester, Minn., Jacksonville, Fla., and Scottsdale, Ariz., Mayo Clinic is dedicated to providing comprehensive diagnoses, accurate answers and effective treatments.

With this depth of medical knowledge, experience and expertise, Mayo Clinic occupies an unparalleled position as a health information resource. Since 1983, Mayo Clinic has published reliable health information for millions of consumers through award-winning newsletters, books and online services. Revenue from the publishing activities supports Mayo Clinic programs, including medical education and research.

Editorial staff

Medical Editor in Chief
Maria·Collazo-Clavell, M.D.

Managing Editor
Elizabeth Davies

Publisher
Sara Gilliland

Editor in Chief
Books and Newsletters
Christopher Frye

Research Manager
Deirdre Herman

Research Librarians
Anthony Cook
Dana Gerberi
Michelle Hewlett

Copy Editing and
Proofreading
Miranda Attlesey
Donna Hanson

Indexing
Larry Harrison

Contributing Writers
Nancy Boudreau
Lee Engfer
Rebecca Gonzalez-Campoy
Tamara Kuhn
Stephen Miller

Creative Director
Daniel Brevick

Designer
Craig King

Illustration
Christopher Srnka

Medical Illustration
Michael King
M. Alice McKinney

Photography
Joseph Kane
Richard Madsen
Randy Ziegler

Administrative Assistants
Beverly Steele
Terri Zanto Strausbauch

Contributing editors and reviewers

Darryl Barnes, M.D.
Ananda Basu, M.D.
Susan Bjornsen, R.N.
M. Regina Castro, M.D.
Diana Dean, M.D.
Andrew Good, M.D.
Sharonne Hayes, M.D.
William Isley, M.D.
Carrie Krieger, Pharm.D.
Yogish Kudva, M.B.B.S.
Edward Laskowski, M.D.
James Levine, M.D., Ph.D.

Aida Lteif, M.D.
M. Molly McMahon, M.D.
Victor Montori, M.D.
Lance Mynderse, M.D.
Jennifer Nelson, R.D.
Robert Rizza, M.D.
W. Frederick Schwenk, M.D.
Steven Smith, M.D.
Peter Tebben, M.D.
Adrian Vella, M.D.
Karen Wallevand
Carol Willett, R.D.

Preface

I f you're reading *Mayo Clinic on Managing Diabetes,* chances are that you or someone close to you has diabetes or is at risk of getting the disease. Diabetes is serious — and increasingly common. But today, more than ever, doctors know what it takes to control diabetes so that you or your loved one can live a healthy and productive life. One thing is certain, successful management of diabetes requires your active involvement on the health care team and a lifelong commitment.

In this second edition, you'll find the latest guidelines on diagnosis and management, as well as valuable self-care tips. You'll learn how diabetes can lead to heart and blood vessel disease and other serious complications, and you'll receive guidance on how to reduce these risks.

Read the latest essential advice on how to manage diabetes — monitoring blood sugar, eating a healthy diet, maintaining a healthy weight, and getting physically active. And you'll learn about various types of insulin and medications, including new drugs, with summary charts for quick comparison. If you're thinking about organ transplantation, our expanded chapter on this topic will provide helpful information.

The section on pregnancy explains how to protect your health and that of your baby. If your child has diabetes, read the new chapter on diabetes in children and adolescents. You'll learn practical tips, from recognizing signs and symptoms, to involving your child in diabetes care, to dealing with emotional issues.

Whether you're reading this book for yourself or a loved one, we hope these strategies, along with guidance from your health care team, will help you live life to the fullest.

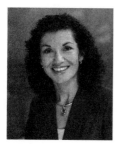

Maria Collazo-Clavell, M.D.
Medical Editor in Chief

Contents

Part 3: Medical Treatments

Part 4: Successful Management

Part 5: Special Issues

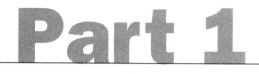

Part 1

The facts

Chapter 1

Understanding diabetes

M aybe your doctor recently broke the news that you have diabetes. Or you've learned that you're at risk of getting the disease. You're worried — afraid of what diabetes will do to you. Will you have to eat tasteless food that has no sugar? Will you have to give yourself daily shots of insulin? Will you eventually face an amputation? Will your diabetes kill you?

For the majority of people with diabetes, the answer to these questions is no. Researchers have learned a great deal about how to diagnose diabetes early and how to control it. Because of these advances, you can live well and not suffer serious complications if you follow your doctor's advice regarding eating, exercise, blood sugar (glucose) monitoring and, when necessary, use of medications.

Due largely to the aging of the American population and the growing number of Americans who are overweight, diabetes is a major health problem in the United States. As your age and weight increase, so does your risk of the most common form of diabetes — type 2. Almost 21 million American adults and children have some form of diabetes. Unfortunately, more than 6 million people don't know it. The reason: Type 2 diabetes can develop gradually over many years and often without symptoms.

Left untreated, diabetes can damage almost every major organ in your body. Diabetes is the sixth leading cause of death and contributes to more than 200,000 deaths in the United States each year. That's why it's important to treat the disease as soon as you discover you have it. Lifestyle changes and medication can help you avoid or reduce the complications of diabetes. If you're willing to do your part, you can enjoy an active and healthy life.

What is diabetes?

The term *diabetes* actually refers to a group of diseases that affect the way your body uses blood glucose, often called blood sugar. Glucose is vital to your health because it's the main source of energy for the cells that make up your muscles and tissues. It's your body's main source of fuel. But if you have diabetes — no matter what type — it means you have too much glucose in your blood, although the reasons why may differ. And too much glucose in your blood can lead to serious problems.

To understand diabetes, first you have to understand how glucose is normally processed.

Normal processing of glucose

Glucose comes from two major sources: the food you eat and your liver. During digestion, glucose is absorbed into your bloodstream. Normally, glucose then enters your body's cells because of the action of insulin.

The hormone insulin comes from your pancreas. When you eat, your pancreas secretes insulin into your bloodstream. As insulin circulates, it acts like a key, unlocking microscopic doors that allow glucose to enter your cells. In this way, insulin lowers the amount of glucose in your bloodstream and prevents it from reaching high levels. As your blood glucose level drops, so does the secretion of insulin from your pancreas.

Your liver acts as a glucose storage and manufacturing center. When the level of insulin in your blood is high, such as after a meal, your liver stores extra glucose as glycogen in case your cells need it later. When your insulin levels are low, for example when you haven't eaten in a while, your liver releases the stored glucose into your bloodstream to keep your glucose level within a normal range.

Normal metabolism

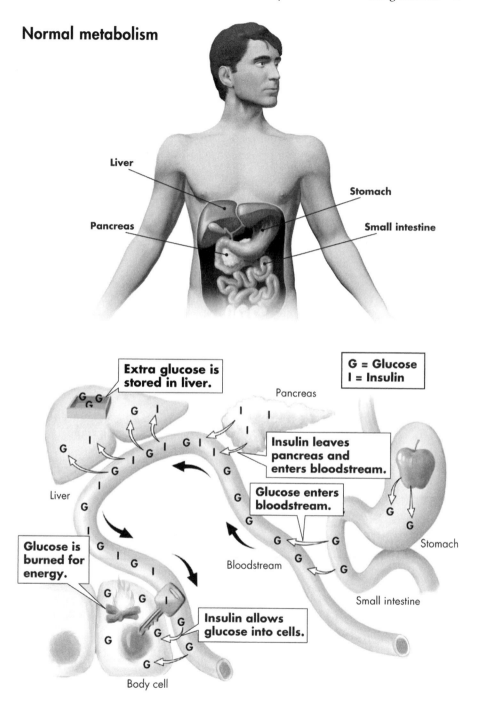

Follow the arrows from right to left: Sugar from the food you eat is converted into glucose, which provides energy to fuel your brain and body. Insulin, released by your pancreas, escorts glucose to your cells (where it's needed for energy) and to your liver (where extra glucose is stored).

When you have diabetes

If you have diabetes, this process doesn't work properly. Instead of being transported into your cells, excess glucose builds up in your bloodstream, and eventually some of it is excreted in your urine. This usually occurs when your pancreas produces little or no insulin, or your cells don't respond properly to insulin, or for both reasons.

The medical term for this condition is diabetes mellitus (MEL-ih-tuhs). Mellitus is a Latin word meaning "honey sweet," referring to the excess sugar in your blood and urine.

Another form of diabetes, called diabetes insipidus (in-SIP-ih-dus), is a rare condition in which the kidneys are unable to conserve water, leading to increased urination and excessive thirst. Rather than an insulin problem, this results from a different hormone disorder. In this book, the term *diabetes* refers to diabetes mellitus.

Types of diabetes

People often think of diabetes as one disease. But glucose can accumulate in your blood for various reasons, resulting in different types of diabetes. The two most common forms are type 1 and type 2.

Type 1

Type 1 diabetes develops when your pancreas makes little if any insulin. Without insulin circulating in your bloodstream, glucose can't get into your cells, so it remains in your blood.

Type 1 diabetes used to be called insulin-dependent diabetes or juvenile diabetes. That's because the disease most often develops when you're a child or a teen, and daily insulin shots are needed to make up for the insulin your body doesn't produce.

But the names insulin-dependent diabetes and juvenile diabetes aren't entirely accurate. Although less common, adults also can develop type 1 diabetes. And the use of insulin isn't limited to people with type 1 disease. People with other forms of diabetes also may need insulin.

Type 1 diabetes is an autoimmune disease, meaning that your own immune system is the culprit. Similar to how it attacks invading viruses or bacteria, your body's infection-fighting system attacks your pancreas, zeroing in on your beta cells, which produce insulin. Researchers aren't certain what causes your immune system to fight your own body, but they believe genetic factors, exposure to certain viruses and diet may be involved. The attacks can dramatically reduce — even entirely wipe out — the insulin-making capacity of your pancreas.

Between 5 percent and 10 percent of people with diabetes have type 1, with the disease occurring almost equally among males and females. The process leading to type 1 diabetes can occur slowly, so it remains undetected for several months or possibly longer. More often, though, symptoms come on quickly, commonly following an illness.

Type 1 diabetes

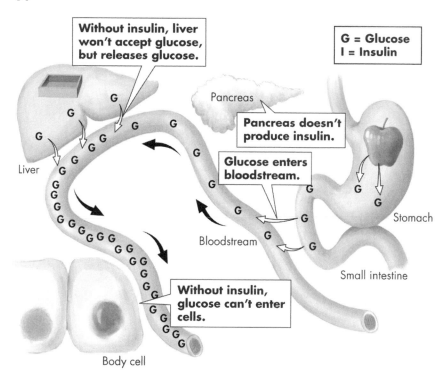

In type 1 diabetes, your pancreas (shown at top) produces little if any insulin. Reading right to left: Sugar from food is converted into glucose. But without insulin to help move glucose into your cells, glucose remains in your bloodstream.

Type 2

Type 2 diabetes is by far the most common form. Ninety percent to 95 percent of people over age 20 who have diabetes have type 2. Like type 1 diabetes, type 2 used to be called by other names: non-insulin-dependent diabetes and adult-onset diabetes. These names reflect that many people with type 2 diabetes don't need insulin shots and that the disease usually develops in adults. As with type 1, these names aren't entirely accurate.

Children and teenagers, as well as adults, can develop type 2 disease. In fact, the incidence of type 2 diabetes in children and adolescents is increasing. In addition, many people with type 2 diabetes need insulin to control their blood glucose.

Type 2 diabetes

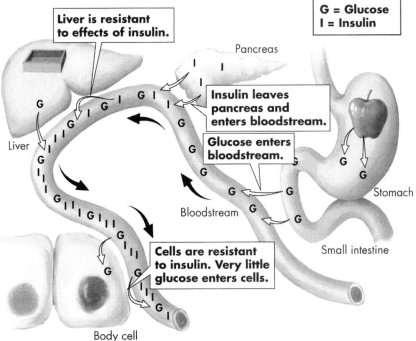

In type 2 diabetes, your pancreas (shown at top) produces insulin. But (reading from right to left) cells don't respond to insulin's effects, causing glucose to remain in your bloodstream after you eat.

Unlike type 1, type 2 diabetes isn't an autoimmune disease. With type 2 diabetes, your pancreas makes insulin, but your cells become resistant to insulin. So insulin can't help move glucose into your cells. As a result, most of the glucose stays in your bloodstream and accumulates.

Exactly why the cells become resistant to insulin is uncertain, although excess weight and fatty tissue seem to be important factors. Most people who develop type 2 diabetes are overweight.

Over time, some people with type 2 diabetes need more insulin. That's because the pancreas may not produce enough insulin, or it may gradually lose its ability to make any insulin. Like people with type 1 diabetes, they become dependent on insulin to control their blood glucose.

Gestational

Gestational diabetes is the name for diabetes that develops during pregnancy. Diabetes can develop temporarily when hormones secreted during pregnancy increase your body's resistance to insulin. This happens in about 4 percent of pregnant women in the United States, although estimates vary.

Gestational diabetes typically develops during the second half of pregnancy — especially in the third trimester — and goes away after the baby is born. But about half of all women who experience gestational diabetes develop type 2 diabetes later in life.

Most pregnant women are screened for gestational diabetes to catch the condition early. If you develop gestational diabetes, being aware of your condition and controlling your blood glucose level throughout your pregnancy can reduce complications for you and your baby. (See "Gestational diabetes," page 198.)

LADA and MODY

Latent autoimmune diabetes of adults (LADA) is a form of type 1 diabetes that develops slowly over many years. LADA is uncommon, but it can be mistaken for type 2 diabetes. Maturity-onset diabetes of the young (MODY) is an uncommon form of type 2 diabetes, caused by a defect in a single gene.

Other causes
A small number of diagnosed cases of diabetes result from conditions or medications that can interfere with the production of insulin or its action. They include: inflammation of the pancreas (pancreatitis), pancreas removal, adrenal or pituitary gland disorders, rare genetic defects, infection, malnutrition or medications used for another disease.

Signs and symptoms

Like many people, because you weren't experiencing any symptoms you may have been shocked to learn that you have diabetes. You felt fine. Often there are no early symptoms. That's especially true with type 2 diabetes. Lack of symptoms and the slow emergence of the disease are the main reasons type 2 diabetes often goes undetected for years.

When symptoms do develop from persistently high blood glucose, they vary. Two classic symptoms that occur in most people with the disease are increased thirst and a frequent need to urinate.

Excessive thirst and increased urination. When you have high levels of glucose in your blood, it overwhelms your kidney's filtering system. Your kidneys can't reabsorb all of the excess glucose, and it's excreted into your urine with fluids drawn from your tissues. This process leads to more frequent urination. As a result, you feel dehydrated. To replace the fluids being drawn out, you're almost constantly drinking water or other beverages.

Flu-like feeling. Symptoms of diabetes, such as fatigue, weakness and loss of appetite, can mimic a viral illness. That's because when you have diabetes and it's not well controlled, the process of using glucose for energy is impaired, affecting your body's function.

Weight loss or gain. Some people, especially those with type 1 diabetes, lose weight before diagnosis. That's because glucose lost through urination leads to calorie loss. More stored fat is used for energy, and muscle tissues may not get enough glucose to generate growth. The weight loss might not be noticeable in people with type 2 diabetes because they tend to be overweight. But in

Diabetes warning signs

Whether you have type 1 or type 2 diabetes, the classic signs and symptoms are:

- Excessive thirst
- Frequent urination

Other signs and symptoms may include:

- Constant hunger
- Unexplained weight loss
- Weight gain (more common in type 2)
- Flu-like symptoms, including weakness and fatigue
- Blurred vision
- Slow-healing cuts or bruises
- Tingling or loss of feeling in hands and feet
- Recurring infections of gums or skin
- Recurring vaginal or bladder infections

most people with type 2, and some people with type 1, diabetes develops after a period of weight gain. Excess weight worsens insulin resistance, leading to an increase in blood glucose levels.

Blurred vision. Excessive glucose in your blood draws the fluid out of the lenses in your eyes, causing them to thin and affecting their ability to focus. Lowering your blood glucose helps restore fluid to your lenses. Your vision may remain blurry for a while as your lenses adjust to the restoration of fluid. But in time vision typically improves.

High blood glucose also can cause the formation of tiny blood vessels in your eyes that can bleed. The blood vessels themselves don't produce symptoms, but bleeding from the vessels can cause dark spots, flashing lights, rings around lights and even blindness. Because diabetes-related eye changes often don't produce symptoms, it's important that you see an eye specialist (ophthalmologist or optometrist) regularly. By dilating your pupils, an eye specialist is able to examine the blood vessels in each retina.

Slow-healing sores or frequent infections. High levels of blood glucose block your body's natural healing process and its ability to fight off infections. For women, bladder and vaginal infections are especially common.

Tingling feet and hands. Excessive glucose in your blood can damage your nerves, which are nourished by your blood. Nerve damage can produce a number of symptoms. The most common nerve-related symptoms are a tingling feeling and a loss of sensation that occurs mainly in your feet and hands. This results from damage to your sensory nerves. You may also experience pain in your extremities — legs, feet, arms and hands — including burning pain.

Red, swollen and tender gums. Diabetes may weaken your mouth's ability to fight germs, increasing your risk of infection in your gums and the bones that hold your teeth in place. Other signs of gum disease include:

- Gums that have pulled away from your teeth, exposing more of your teeth or even part of the root
- Sores or pockets of pus in your gums
- Permanent teeth becoming loose
- Changes in the fit of your dentures

Factors that increase your risk

Perhaps you've heard one of the common myths about diabetes — that it comes from eating too much sugar. Not true. Researchers don't fully understand why some people develop the disease and others don't. It's clear though that your lifestyle and certain health conditions can increase your risk.

Family history. Your chance of developing either type 1 or type 2 diabetes increases if someone in your immediate family has the disease, whether that person is a parent, brother or sister (see the chart on page 20). Genetics plays a role in the disease, but exactly how certain genes may cause diabetes is unknown.

Scientists are studying genes that may be linked to diabetes, but tests are still under development and not available for routine clinical use. Although people who develop diabetes may have inherited a tendency toward the disease, an environmental factor usually triggers this tendency.

Weight. Being overweight or obese is one of the most common risk factors for type 2 diabetes. More than 85 percent of people with type 2 diabetes are overweight or obese.

The more fatty tissue you have, the more resistant your muscle and tissue cells become to your own insulin. This is especially true if your excess weight is concentrated around your abdomen and your body is an apple shape rather than a pear shape, where the weight is mostly on the hips and thighs.

Many people with diabetes who are overweight can improve their blood glucose simply by losing weight. Even small weight loss can have beneficial effects, reducing blood glucose levels or allowing diabetes medications to work better.

Inactivity. The less active you are, the greater your risk of type 2 diabetes. Physical activity helps you control your weight, uses up glucose as energy, makes your cells more sensitive to insulin, increases blood flow and improves circulation.

Exercise also helps build muscle mass. That's important because most of the glucose in your blood is absorbed by your muscles and burns as energy.

Age. Your risk of type 2 diabetes increases as you grow older, especially after age 45. At least one in five Americans age 65 or older has diabetes. Part of the reason is that as people grow older, they tend to become less physically active, lose muscle mass and gain weight.

Recent years, however, have seen a dramatic rise in type 2 diabetes among people in their 30s and 40s. And more children and teenagers are being diagnosed with type 2 diabetes. (See "If your child has diabetes," Chapter 13.)

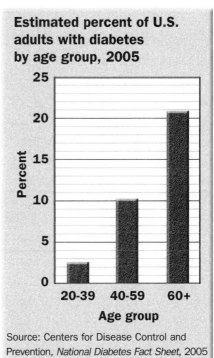

Estimated percent of U.S. adults with diabetes by age group, 2005

Source: Centers for Disease Control and Prevention, *National Diabetes Fact Sheet*, 2005

For 2005, it's estimated that more than 2 percent of adults ages 20 to 39, about 10 percent of adults ages 40 to 59, and almost 21 percent of adults age 60 or older have type 1 or type 2 diabetes.

Metabolic syndrome increases your risk of disease

Although not all experts agree, metabolic syndrome (also called insulin resistance syndrome) is a group of risk factors that make you more likely to develop type 2 diabetes, heart disease and stroke. If you have three or more of the risk factors below, you may be diagnosed with metabolic syndrome.

- **Abdominal obesity:** More than a 35-inch waist for women and more than a 40-inch waist for men*
- **Triglycerides:** 150 mg/dL or above, or drug treatment for high triglycerides
- **HDL cholesterol** (high-density lipoprotein, the "good" kind): Lower than 50 mg/dL for women and lower than 40 mg/dL for men, or drug treatment for low HDL
- **Blood pressure:** Systolic (top number) of 130 mm Hg or above or diastolic (bottom number) of 85 mm Hg or above, or drug treatment for high blood pressure
- **Fasting blood glucose:** 100 mg/dL or higher, or drug treatment for high blood glucose

If you think that you have metabolic syndrome, talk with your doctor about tests that can help determine this. Healthy eating, achieving a healthy weight and increasing your level of physical activity can help combat metabolic syndrome and play a role in preventing diabetes and other serious diseases.

*For Asian Americans: Over a 31-inch waist for women and over a 35-inch waist for men

Source: American Heart Association/National Heart, Lung, and Blood Institute, 2005

Race. About 7 percent of the U.S. population has diabetes. Although it's unclear why, people of certain races are more likely to develop diabetes than others. Type 1 diabetes is more common in white Americans than in black Americans, Hispanic Americans or other ethnic groups.

However, if you're a black American or Hispanic American, you're about one and a half times more likely to have type 2 diabetes than someone who's white. If you're an American Indian or Alaska Native, your risk of type 2 diabetes more than doubles compared with whites. Asian Americans and Pacific Islanders also have a higher risk of type 2 diabetes than white Americans do.

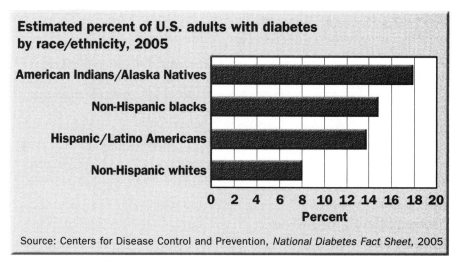

Estimated percent of U.S. adults with diabetes by race/ethnicity, 2005

Source: Centers for Disease Control and Prevention, *National Diabetes Fact Sheet*, 2005

For 2005, it's estimated that 8 percent of non-Hispanic white adults (age 20 and older) have type 1 or type 2 diabetes. But the percentage of adults with diabetes is higher in other groups, affecting almost 18 percent of American Indians and Alaska Natives, almost 15 percent of non-Hispanic blacks, and almost 14 percent of Hispanic/Latino Americans.

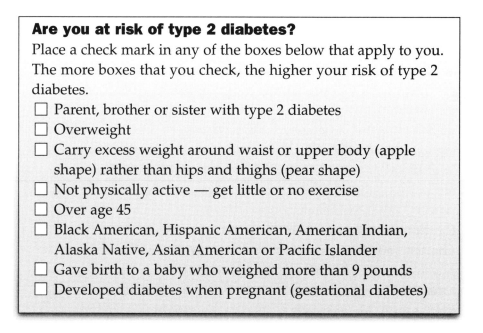

Are you at risk of type 2 diabetes?

Place a check mark in any of the boxes below that apply to you. The more boxes that you check, the higher your risk of type 2 diabetes.

☐ Parent, brother or sister with type 2 diabetes
☐ Overweight
☐ Carry excess weight around waist or upper body (apple shape) rather than hips and thighs (pear shape)
☐ Not physically active — get little or no exercise
☐ Over age 45
☐ Black American, Hispanic American, American Indian, Alaska Native, Asian American or Pacific Islander
☐ Gave birth to a baby who weighed more than 9 pounds
☐ Developed diabetes when pregnant (gestational diabetes)

Tests to detect diabetes

Many people first learn they have diabetes through blood tests done for another condition or as part of a complete physical exam. Most doctors don't screen for diabetes during routine visits. Sometimes, though, a doctor may test specifically for diabetes if he or she suspects the disease, based on symptoms or risk factors. Any one of several tests may indicate whether you have diabetes, but some are more accurate than others.

Fasting blood glucose test

The amount of glucose in your blood naturally fluctuates, but within a narrow range. Your blood glucose level is typically highest after a meal and lowest after an overnight fast. The preferred way to test your blood glucose is after you've fasted overnight or for at least eight hours. Blood is drawn from a vein and sent to a lab for evaluation.

A fasting blood glucose level under 100 milligrams of glucose per deciliter of blood (mg/dL) is considered normal. If your glucose level measures from 100 to 125 mg/dL, you have impaired fasting glucose, commonly referred to as prediabetes. Prediabetes shouldn't be taken lightly. It's a sign that you're at high risk of developing the disease and that you should see your doctor regularly and take steps to control your glucose.

If — after two tests — your glucose results are 126 mg/dL or higher after at least eight hours of fasting, you have diabetes. If your blood glucose is above 200 mg/dL, with symptoms of diabetes, a second test may not be necessary to reach the diagnosis.

Random blood glucose test

This test may be a part of the routine blood work done during a physical exam. Using a needle inserted into a vein, blood is drawn for a variety of laboratory tests. This is done without any special preparation on your part, such as an overnight fast.

Even if you've recently eaten and your blood glucose is at its peak, the level shouldn't be above 200 mg/dL. If it is, and if you have symptoms of diabetes, you can expect a diagnosis of diabetes.

Understanding your fasting glucose test results

If you have symptoms that suggest diabetes, ask your doctor for a fasting blood glucose test. Have a baseline test by age 45. If your results are normal, get tested every three years. If you have prediabetes, have this test at least once a year. If you're overweight with one or more additional risk factors for diabetes, get tested at a younger age and more frequently.

Glucose level	Indicates
Under 100 mg/dL	Normal
100 to 125 mg/dL	Prediabetes*
126 mg/dL or higher on two separate tests	Diabetes

mg/dL = Milligrams of glucose per deciliter of blood

*Prediabetes means that you're at high risk of developing diabetes.

Oral glucose tolerance test

This test is less commonly used today because other tests are less expensive and easier to administer. An oral glucose tolerance test requires that you visit a lab or your doctor's office after at least an eight-hour fast. There you drink about 8 ounces of a sweet liquid that contains a lot of sugar — about 75 grams.

Your blood glucose is measured before you drink the liquid, then after one hour, and again after two hours. If you have diabetes, your blood glucose rises more than normal. If your blood glucose reaches between 140 and 199 mg/dL after two hours, you have impaired glucose tolerance, another prediabetes condition. If your blood glucose is 200 mg/dL or above after two hours, you have diabetes.

For this test to be accurate, you should follow your usual diet and be in good health with no other illness — not even a cold. You also should be relatively active and not taking medication that could affect your blood glucose level. Doctors often use a modified version of this test to check pregnant women for gestational diabetes.

Can diabetes be prevented?

At this time, there is no way to prevent type 1 diabetes. But a major clinical study shows that lifestyle changes can prevent type 2 diabetes in many people. The National Institutes of Health's Diabetes Prevention Program involved more than 3,200 people from across the United States who were followed for almost three years. Almost half of the participants were from racial or ethnic groups at higher risk of developing diabetes.

All participants were overweight and had prediabetes. They were randomly assigned to one of three groups:

1. Group 1 received intensive training on a healthy diet (low-fat and low-calorie), moderately intense physical activity (such as brisk walking) 150 minutes a week, and behavior modification. They aimed to lose 7 percent of their weight.
2. Group 2 took 850 milligrams (mg) of an oral diabetes drug called metformin (Glucophage) twice a day.
3. Group 3 took inactive pills (placebos) instead of a drug.

Results of the Diabetes Prevention Program

The results of the Diabetes Prevention Program (see box on next page) were so successful that the study was ended a year early. It showed that many people may prevent or delay the onset of type 2 diabetes by eating a nutritious diet that's low in fat and calories, achieving modest weight loss and keeping physically active. Treatment with metformin can also reduce the incidence of diabetes in high-risk people, although the lifestyle intervention was more effective.

Reducing your risk

If you've already been diagnosed with diabetes — no matter what type — you can greatly reduce your risk of serious complications by healthy eating (Chapter 4), achieving a healthy weight (Chapter 5) and getting more physically active (Chapter 6).

Diabetes Prevention Program results

Treament group	Risk of diabetes reduced by*	Comments
Group 1: Lifestyle (healthy diet and moderately intense physical activity)	58% for entire group 71% for those age 60 and older	Half of the lifestyle group lost 7% or more of their weight within six months.
Group 2: Metformin (oral drug for diabetes, 850 mg twice a day)	31% (overall, about half as effective as the lifestyle group results)	Metformin was most effective in people ages 25 to 44 years and in those at least 60 pounds overweight. It was almost ineffective in people 60 years and older or those who were less overweight.

*Compared with an inactive pill (placebo)

Based on Diabetes Prevention Program Research Group, "Reduction in the incidence of type 2 diabetes with lifestyle intervention or metformin," *The New England Journal of Medicine*, Feb. 7, 2002

Questions and answers

Is there a cure for diabetes?
No. Researchers continue looking for ways to cure diabetes, but now doctors can only treat the disease, not cure it.

How long do most people have diabetes before it's diagnosed?
Because type 1 diabetes generally occurs more suddenly and severely, it's usually diagnosed within a few months. People with type 2 diabetes, however, may have the disease for several years before it's diagnosed. But, as noted earlier, you can take steps to prevent type 2 diabetes through healthy lifestyle changes.

What is insulin resistance?

Insulin resistance means your body can't use insulin properly, causing your blood glucose levels to rise above normal. This increases your chances of developing type 2 diabetes as well as heart and blood vessel disease. If you already have diabetes, you probably had insulin resistance long before your diagnosis.

Insulin resistance is often a part of the metabolic syndrome (explained on page 14), and risk factors are similar. Many other conditions are linked with insulin resistance. For example, women with polycystic ovary syndrome (PCOS) — a hormone disorder that can cause infertility — are also at risk of insulin resistance. Many people can prevent or reverse insulin resistance by healthy eating, losing weight and increasing physical activity.

If I have a close relative with diabetes — a parent, brother or sister — what are my chances of getting the disease?

For reasons that aren't well understood, your risk of developing diabetes varies, as shown below. Note that family history (which relates to both learned behavior and genetics) and lifestyle seem to play a larger role in the development of type 2 diabetes. Many people with type 1 diabetes have no known family history.

How does family history affect your risk of diabetes?

Type 1		Type 2*	
Relative with diabetes	**Your estimated risk**	**Relative with diabetes**	**Your estimated risk**
Mother	1% to 5%	Mother	5% to 20%
Father	5% to 15%	Father	5% to 20%
Both parents	10% to 25%	Both parents	25% to 50%
Brother or sister	5% to 10%	Brother or sister	25% to 50%
Identical twin	25% to 50%	Identical twin	60% to 75%

*Having a healthy diet, maintaining a healthy weight and exercising regularly can substantially lower your overall risk of type 2 diabetes.

Source: Based on a review of recent medical journal articles and textbooks

Chapter 2

The dangers of uncontrolled diabetes

Diabetes is often easy to ignore, especially in the early stages. You're feeling fine. Your body seems to be working well. No symptoms. No problem. Right?

Not even close. While you're doing nothing, the excess sugar (glucose) in your blood is eroding the very fabric of your body, threatening major organs, including your heart, nerves, eyes and kidneys. You may not feel the effects right away, but eventually you will.

Compared with people who don't have diabetes, when you have diabetes you're:

- Two to four times more likely to die of a heart attack
- Two to four times more likely to have a stroke

And in U.S. adults, diabetes is the leading cause of:

- Blindness in people ages 20 to 74
- Kidney failure (end-stage renal disease)
- Limb amputation

Researchers are making great progress in understanding what triggers complications of diabetes and how to manage or prevent them. Several studies show that if you keep your blood glucose close to normal, you can dramatically reduce your risks of complications. And it's never too late to start. As soon as you begin managing your glucose level, you may slow the progression of complications and reduce your chances of developing more health problems.

If you have diabetes, you need to be on the alert for emergencies as well as long-term complications.

Medical emergencies

Medical emergencies require immediate attention as explained in each section below.

Low blood glucose (hypoglycemia)

Low blood glucose — a level below 70 milligrams of glucose per deciliter of blood (mg/dL) — is called hypoglycemia (hi-po-gli-SEE-mee-uh). This condition basically results from too much insulin and too little glucose in your blood. If your blood glucose level drops too low — for example, below 50 mg/dL — this could result in unconsciousness, a condition sometimes called insulin shock or coma.

Hypoglycemia, also called an insulin reaction, is most common among people taking insulin. It can also occur in people taking oral medications that enhance the release of insulin.

Your blood glucose level can drop for many reasons, such as:
- Skipping or delaying a meal
- Eating too few carbohydrates
- Exercising longer or more strenuously than normal
- Having too much insulin from not adjusting your medication when you have changes in your blood glucose

What are the signs and symptoms?
Signs and symptoms of hypoglycemia vary, depending on how low your blood glucose level drops.
Early signs and symptoms:
- Sweating
- Shakiness
- Visual disturbances
- Nervousness
- Headache
- Fast heartbeat
- Weakness
- Hunger
- Dizziness
- Irritability
- Nausea
- Cold, clammy skin

Later signs and symptoms: (typically occurs with a blood glucose level below 40 mg/dL)

- Slurred speech
- Drunken-like behavior
- Drowsiness
- Confusion

Emergency signs and symptoms:

- Convulsions
- Unconsciousness (coma), which can be fatal

What should you do?

As soon as you suspect that your blood glucose is low, check your glucose level. If it's below 70 mg/dL, eat or drink something that will raise your level quickly. Good examples include:

- Hard candy, equal to about five LifeSavers
- A regular — not diet — soft drink
- Half a cup of fruit juice
- Glucose tablets (nonprescription pills made especially for treating low blood glucose)

If after 15 minutes you continue to experience symptoms, repeat the treatment. If they still don't go away, contact your doctor or call for emergency assistance.

If you lose consciousness or for some other reason can't swallow, you'll need an injection of glucagon, a fast-acting hormone that stimulates the release of glucose into your blood. Teach your close

---

Do you miss the early warning signs of hypoglycemia?

Some people who have had diabetes for several years don't experience early signs and symptoms of low blood glucose, such as shakiness or nervousness. That's because chemical changes from long-standing diabetes may mask the symptoms or keep them from occurring.

With this condition, called hypoglycemia unawareness, you may not realize your blood glucose is low until later signs and symptoms, such as confusion or slurred speech, set in. If you're concerned about hypoglycemia unawareness, work with your health care team to identify circumstances that put you at risk of hypoglycemia and discuss ways to help prevent it.

friends and family members how to give you the shot in case of an emergency. Also tell them to call 911 (or your local emergency number if your area isn't covered by 911) if the shot doesn't help and you don't regain consciousness quickly.

A glucagon emergency kit includes the medication and a syringe. The shot is easy to administer and is generally given in an arm, or buttock, or thigh or the abdomen. The medication starts to act in about five minutes. If you take insulin, you should have a glucagon kit with or near you at all times. Many people have several kits and keep one in each of their vehicles, at home, at work and in a purse or sports bag.

What is hyperglycemia?

The medical term for high blood glucose (anything above normal) is hyperglycemia. Whether you have prediabetes or diabetes, you have hyperglycemia. The key is to make sure that your blood glucose doesn't get out of control.

If you have diabetes, regularly testing your blood glucose and keeping it in the target range that your health care team recommended can help prevent serious hyperglycemia. If hyperglycemia isn't dealt with early, it can lead to life-threatening problems, such as hyperosmolar hyperglycemic state (HHS) or diabetic ketoacidosis (DKA).

Hyperosmolar hyperglycemic state (HHS)

When your blood glucose reaches a dangerously high level, your blood actually becomes thick and syrupy. This condition, called hyperosmolar (hi-pur-oz-MO-lur) hyperglycemic state (HHS), may occur when your blood glucose level gets over 600 mg/dL. Your cells can't absorb this much glucose, so the glucose passes from your blood into your urine. This triggers a filtering process that draws tremendous amounts of fluid from your body and results in dehydration, a condition caused by too much water loss.

HHS is most common in people with type 2 diabetes, especially people who don't monitor their blood glucose or who don't know they have diabetes. It can occur in people with diabetes who are taking high-dose steroids or drugs that increase urination. It also may be brought on by an infection (such as a urinary tract infection or pneumonia), illness, stress, drinking too much alcohol or drug abuse. Older adults with diabetes who don't get enough fluids are also at risk of HHS.

What are the signs and symptoms?
Signs and symptoms of HHS include:

- Excessive thirst
- Dry mouth
- Frequent urination
- Dehydration
- Weakness
- Leg cramps
- Rapid pulse
- Seizures
- Confusion
- Coma

What should you do?
Check your blood glucose level. If it's more than 350 mg/dL, call your doctor for advice. If it's 500 mg/dL or higher, see a doctor immediately. This is an emergency situation — have someone else drive.

Emergency treatment can correct the problem within hours. You'll likely receive intravenous fluids to restore water to your tissues, and short-acting insulin to help your tissue cells absorb glucose. Without prompt treatment, the condition can be fatal.

High level of ketones (diabetic ketoacidosis)

When you don't get enough insulin over a period of time, your muscle cells become so starved for energy that your body takes emergency measures and breaks down fat. As your body transforms the fat into energy, it produces blood acids known as ketones. A buildup of ketones in the blood is called ketoacidosis (kee-toe-ass-ih-DOE-sis). Diabetic ketoacidosis (DKA) is a dangerous condition that can be fatal if untreated.

DKA is more common in people with type 1 diabetes. It can be caused by skipping some of your shots or not raising your insulin dose to adjust for a rise in your blood glucose level.

Extreme stress or illness, which can occur in people with either type 1 or type 2 diabetes, also may cause DKA. When you develop an infection, your body produces certain hormones, such as adrenaline, to help fight off the problem. Unfortunately, these hormones also work against insulin. Sometimes the two causes occur together. You get sick or overstressed, and you forget to take your insulin.

In people who are unaware they have diabetes, DKA can be the first sign of the disease. Early symptoms of DKA can be confused with the flu, which may delay appropriate medical attention.

What are the signs and symptoms?
As the level of ketones in your blood rises, you may experience:

- High blood glucose
- Dry mouth
- Excessive thirst
- Frequent urination

Later signs and symptoms of DKA include:

- Fatigue
- Nausea
- Vomiting
- Abdominal pain
- Shallow breathing
- Sweet, fruity odor on your breath
- Blurry vision
- Confusion
- Loss of appetite
- Weight loss
- Weakness
- Drowsiness

What should you do?
Check your ketone level if you experience any of the signs or symptoms above or whenever your blood glucose is persistently over 250 mg/dL. It's a good idea to also check your ketone level if you're generally feeling sick or especially stressed.

You can buy a ketones test kit at a drugstore or pharmacy and do the test at home. Most kits use chemically treated strips that you dip into your urine. When you have high amounts of ketones in your blood, excess ketones are excreted in your urine. Test strips in the kit change color according to the level of ketones in your urine: low, moderate or high.

If the color on your test strip shows a moderate or a high ketone level, call your doctor right away for advice on how much insulin to take, and drink plenty of water to prevent dehydration. If you have a high ketone level and you can't reach your doctor, go to a hospital emergency room. Left untreated, DKA can lead to a coma and possibly death.

DKA requires emergency medical treatment, which involves replenishing lost fluids through intravenous (IV) lines. Insulin, which may be combined with glucose, is injected into an IV line so that your body will stop making ketones. Gradually, your blood glucose level is brought back to normal. Adjusting your blood glucose too quickly can produce swelling in your brain. But this complication appears to be more common in children, especially those with newly diagnosed diabetes.

You'll likely need a hospital stay if:
• You can't control your blood glucose
• You become confused
• You're unable to eat or drink

Long-term complications

Long-term diabetes complications develop gradually and may lead to other disabling or life-threatening diseases.

Heart and blood vessel disease

Heart and blood vessel disease (cardiovascular disease) is the leading cause of death among people with diabetes. Diabetes can damage your major arteries as well as your small blood vessels, making it easier for fatty deposits (plaques) to form in arteries, a condition called atherosclerosis (ath-ur-o-skluh-ROE-sis). This narrowing of arteries causes an increased risk of a heart attack, stroke and other disorders caused by impaired circulation.

Coronary artery disease
Coronary artery disease is caused by atherosclerosis in blood vessels that feed your heart (coronary arteries). Over time, fatty deposits can narrow your coronary arteries, so less oxygen-rich

Diabetes promotes development of atherosclerosis

Your arteries can become narrowed or blocked by a complex process called atherosclerosis.

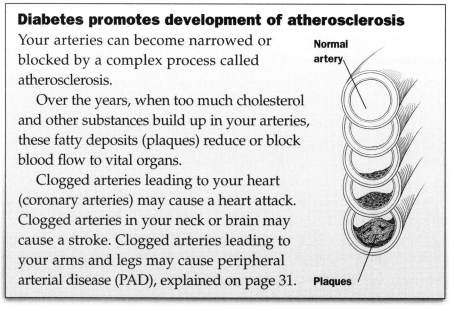

Normal artery

Plaques

Over the years, when too much cholesterol and other substances build up in your arteries, these fatty deposits (plaques) reduce or block blood flow to vital organs.

Clogged arteries leading to your heart (coronary arteries) may cause a heart attack. Clogged arteries in your neck or brain may cause a stroke. Clogged arteries leading to your arms and legs may cause peripheral arterial disease (PAD), explained on page 31.

blood flows to your heart muscle. Atherosclerosis develops slowly and silently over decades, often going unnoticed. Once a blockage is severe enough, heart muscle can be damaged due to a lack of oxygen (ischemia), causing a heart attack.

What are the signs and symptoms of coronary artery disease?

Signs and symptoms of coronary artery disease vary, as does severity, depending on the extent of the disease and the individual. In its early stages, coronary artery disease often produces no symptoms. Later on, you may experience symptoms that limit your ability to perform your usual tasks, such as:

- Shortness of breath
- Fatigue
- Rapid or irregular heartbeats (palpitations)

Or you may have warning signs of a heart attack.

Heart attack. You could be having a heart attack if you have any of these signs or symptoms:

- Pressure, fullness or squeezing pain in the center of your chest for more than a few minutes
- Pain extending beyond your chest to your shoulder, arm, back, or even your teeth and jaw
- Increasing or prolonged episodes of chest pain

- Prolonged pain in the upper abdomen
- Shortness of breath
- Sweating
- Impending sense of doom
- Lightheadedness
- Fainting
- Nausea and vomiting

If you think you're having a heart attack, immediately call 911 (or your local emergency number if your area isn't covered by 911).

Damage to your heart from a heart attack increases your risk of developing heart failure over time, with symptoms such as shortness of breath and swelling in your legs, ankles and feet.

Silent heart attacks

If you have diabetes, you're at particular risk of silent (asymptomatic) heart attacks — heart attacks without typical symptoms. Diabetes can damage nerves that transmit chest pain, which typically accompanies a heart attack. Without pain sensations, you may be unaware that a heart attack is occurring.

Even without diabetes, many women and older adults often don't have the classic early warning signs of a heart attack, such as chest pain. Still, the more signs and symptoms you have, the more likely you're having a heart attack.

How is coronary artery disease treated?

To improve blood flow to the heart muscle and relieve symptoms or to help prevent coronary artery disease, your doctor may recommend drug therapy such as:

Aspirin. Low-dose daily aspirin can reduce the tendency of your blood to clot, which may help prevent blockage of your coronary arteries. But daily aspirin isn't safe for everyone — check with your doctor.

Cholesterol-lowering drugs. Cholesterol is a large part of the deposits that can narrow heart arteries. Lowering cholesterol plays a critical role in the prevention and treatment of coronary artery disease. Most people with diabetes will require cholesterol-lowering medications to achieve the recommended cholesterol levels.

Blood pressure drugs. Lowering your blood pressure eases the workload on your heart and improves blood flow in your arteries.

Other drugs. Depending on your specific type of coronary artery disease, other kinds of drugs may be recommended.

Your doctor may recommend a cardiac catheterization (kath-et-er-ih-ZA-shun). During this procedure, dye is injected into the blood vessels of your heart. The dye, visible by X-ray, shows where and how many blockages are present. If warranted, your doctor may recommend angioplasty and stenting to open arteries, or surgery to bypass clogged arteries.

Stroke

A stroke occurs when the blood supply to a part of your brain is interrupted or severely reduced and brain tissue is deprived of oxygen and nutrients. Within a few minutes to a few hours, brain cells begin to die. The interruption can be from a clogged or blocked artery (ischemic stroke) or from a leaking or ruptured artery (hemorrhagic stroke). Ischemic (is-KEE-mik) stroke is more common.

What are the signs and symptoms of stroke?

The most common signs and symptoms include:

- Sudden numbness, weakness or paralysis of the face, arm or leg — usually on one side of the body
- Loss of speech, or trouble talking or understanding speech
- Sudden blurred, double or decreased vision
- Dizziness, loss of balance or loss of coordination
- A sudden, severe or unusual headache, possibly with a stiff neck, facial pain, pain between the eyes, vomiting or altered consciousness
- Confusion, or problems with memory, spatial orientation or perception

If you think you're having a stroke, immediately call 911 or your local emergency number.

How is stroke treated?

Immediate treatment for ischemic stroke tries to improve blood flow. This may include injection of a clot-busting drug such as tissue plasminogen activator (TPA) or the use of the blood-thinners heparin or warfarin (Coumadin). Immediate treatment for hemorrhagic stroke aims to stop the bleeding from the artery leak or rupture, which may require surgery. Long-term treatment depends on the extent of the damage and focuses on recovering any lost function (such as the ability to speak) and preventing future strokes.

Peripheral arterial disease (PAD)

With PAD, the arteries supplying blood to your limbs — more commonly your legs — become clogged or partially blocked due to atherosclerosis. If you have PAD, you may also have clogged arteries in other parts of your body. PAD is serious — it increases your risk of a heart attack, stroke and lower limb amputation.

What are the signs and symptoms of PAD?

Initially, impaired blood flow can cause pain, cramping or fatigue in your legs or buttocks when walking. These signs and symptoms go away with rest. If you have more severe PAD, you may experience a burning or aching pain in your feet or toes when you're resting. You may also have leg or foot sores that don't heal.

How is PAD treated?

Treatment involves slowing the progression of atherosclerosis and improving blood flow to the affected tissues. Common recommendations include medications to control cholesterol and high blood pressure, and possibly surgery to bypass obstructed vessels.

Prevention of heart and blood vessel disease

Changing your lifestyle remains the single most effective way to prevent the development and stop the progression of heart and blood vessel disease. Follow these recommendations and learn more about them in upcoming chapters:

- Don't smoke
- Control your blood pressure
- Control your cholesterol
- Eat a heart-healthy diet
- Exercise regularly
- Maintain a healthy weight
- Get regular medical checkups
- Manage stress

Nerve damage (neuropathy)

Nerve damage, also called neuropathy (noo-ROP-uh-thee), is a common long-term complication of diabetes. You have a complex network of nerves that runs throughout your body, connecting your brain to muscles, skin and other organs. Through these nerves, your brain senses pain, controls your muscles and performs automatic tasks such as breathing and digestion. High levels of blood glucose can damage these delicate nerves. Excess glucose is thought to weaken the walls of tiny blood vessels (capillaries) that nourish your nerves.

Diabetic neuropathy affects about half of all people with diabetes. Sometimes the results can be painful and disabling. More often the symptoms are mild.

What are the signs and symptoms?

There are many kinds of nerve damage:

- Damage to your sensory nerves may leave you unable to detect sensations such as pain, warmth, coolness and texture.
- Damage to your autonomic nerves can increase your heart rate and perspiration level. In men, such damage can interfere with their ability to have an erection (see chapter 12).
- Damage to nerves that control your muscles may leave you with weakened muscles and loss of strength.

Most commonly, diabetes damages the sensory nerves in your legs, and less often, your arms. You may experience any of these symptoms, which often begin at the tips of your toes, fingers, or both and — over a period of months or years — gradually spread upward:

- A tingling feeling, numbness, pain or a combination of these sensations
- Burning pain that comes and goes
- Stabbing or aching pain that's worse at night
- A crawling sensation

Doctors often can detect sensory nerve damage. If, for example, the nerves in a toe are damaged, you won't be able to feel a light pinprick or the vibration of a tuning fork held against the toe. Left untreated, symptoms of decreased sensation can progress, putting you at high risk of injuring your feet without realizing it. Minor injuries, when not recognized early, can lead to bigger problems, such as ulcerations and even amputations in people with diabetes. (See "Care for your feet," page 169.)

How is it treated?
Good blood glucose control may reduce your symptoms. To help relieve pain, your doctor may prescribe a pain reliever or other medications that also can reduce pain.

Another treatment for nerve-related pain is a nonprescription cream called capsaicin (Axsain, Capzasin-P, Zostrix), which contains hot pepper extract. When you rub the cream on your skin, it helps block pain sensations. Relief usually begins within two to four weeks after you start using the cream. To keep the pain from returning, you need to apply the cream daily. Other therapies for pain relief include acupuncture, biofeedback and relaxation techniques.

Because your sensation to hot and cold temperatures may be reduced, take care not to burn yourself when bathing or using an electric blanket or heating pad. Also guard against frostbite in cold temperatures.

Kidney disease (nephropathy)

Each of your kidneys has about a million nephrons. A nephron is a tiny filtering unit with tiny blood vessels (capillaries) that remove waste from your blood and send it to your urine. Diabetes can damage this delicate filtering system, often before you notice any symptoms. Up to 30 percent of people with diabetes eventually develop kidney disease, called nephropathy (nuh-FROP-uh-thee). The longer you have diabetes, the higher your risk of kidney damage.

What are the signs and symptoms?
In its early stages, kidney disease produces few symptoms. Generally, damage is extensive before these signs and symptoms occur:
- Swelling of the ankles, feet and hands
- Shortness of breath
- High blood pressure
- Confusion or difficulty concentrating

- Poor appetite
- Metallic taste in your mouth
- Fatigue

How is it treated?

Treatment depends on how advanced the disease is. For early disease, keeping your blood glucose level near normal can prevent your condition from getting worse, and possibly improve it.

Excellent control of your blood pressure is also critically important, as noted in the section on heart and blood vessel disease. Angiotensin-converting enzyme (ACE) inhibitors or drugs called angiotensin receptor blockers (ARBs) are often used because they can help slow the progression of kidney disease and help lower your blood pressure. Another option is to eat a low-protein diet, which seems to reduce the workload of your kidneys. But consult your doctor or dietitian before making changes to your diet.

Treatment for severe damage, known as kidney failure or end-stage renal disease, includes kidney dialysis or a kidney transplant. During kidney dialysis your blood is funneled through a machine that removes waste from it. (See "Dialysis and transplantation," Chapter 9.)

Diabetes is the nation's leading cause of kidney failure. For unclear reasons, kidney failure is escalating among certain races. Black Americans, Hispanic Americans (especially Mexican Americans) and American Indians have a higher incidence of type 2 diabetes than white Americans do.

Eye damage (retinopathy)

Many tiny vessels nourish the back part of your eye, called the retina. These blood vessels are often among the first to be damaged by high blood glucose. This damage is called diabetic retinopathy (ret-ih-NOP-uh-thee).

Nearly everyone with type 1 diabetes and more than six out of 10 people with type 2 diabetes develop some form of eye damage by the time they've had diabetes for 20 years. Most people experience only mild vision problems. For others, the effects are more severe, including blindness. Diabetes is the leading cause of blindness in adults in the United States. Each year thousands of people lose their sight from diabetes.

There are two types of diabetic retinopathy:

Nonproliferative. This form is mild and the most common. Blood vessels in your retina become weak and may swell or develop bulges or fatty deposits. The condition generally doesn't affect your vision unless some of the swollen vessels are in the tiny portion of your retina called the macula, which is responsible for your sharpest vision.

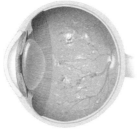

In nonproliferative diabetic retinopathy, the walls of blood vessels in the retina weaken. The vessel walls develop tiny bulges or pouches.

Proliferative. When tiny blood vessels in the retina are damaged, they can bleed or close off. New and fragile blood vessels may form (proliferate) in the retina, and they too may bleed. If this bleeding is heavy or occurs in certain areas of the eye, it can damage your retina, leading to blindness. New blood vessels also can form scar tissue that can push or pull on your retina and distort your vision.

Proliferative retinopathy may require special treatment by an ophthalmologist. To protect your vision, it's important to catch the disease early so that it can be treated.

What are the signs and symptoms?

Early diabetic retinopathy often produces few, if any, visual symptoms or pain. As the damage gradually becomes more severe, these symptoms may develop:

- "Spiders," "cobwebs" or tiny specks floating in your vision
- Blurred vision
- A dark or empty spot in the center of your vision
- Dark streaks or a red film that blocks vision
- Flashes of light
- Poor night vision
- Vision loss

How is it treated?

Regular eye examinations can identify problems early before permanent damage occurs. Treatment may include a laser procedure to seal weak blood vessels and stop them from leaking. In most cases only one eye is treated at a time. You may need several treatments, which are usually painless. If bleeding into the middle of an eye occurs, you may need a surgical procedure to remove the blood and replace it with a clear fluid that allows light to pass through to the retina.

A displaced or detached retina from buildup of scar tissue generally requires surgery to position the retina in place. Your vision may take several months to improve and, in some cases, may never fully return.

Increased risk of infection

High blood glucose impairs the function of your immune cells to fight off invading germs and bacteria, putting you at higher risk of infection. Your mouth, gums, lungs, skin, feet, bladder and genital area are common infection sites.

High blood glucose can also damage those nerves that would otherwise alert you to a potential infection. An example is your bladder. Damage to nerves that control bladder sensations may fail to alert you that your bladder is full. As a result of constantly being overstretched, your bladder may lose its muscle tone and its ability to empty completely. Bacteria may grow in the remaining urine, causing an infection.

What are the signs and symptoms?

Sign and symptoms of infection vary, depending on its location. A low-grade fever is common with many infections. If the infection is in your gums, you may experience red and bleeding gums. A bladder infection typically causes frequent urination, an urgency to urinate and a burning sensation while urinating. A common symptom of a vaginal infection is itching in the genital area. For a foot wound, redness around the injury site or an accumulation of pus often is a warning of an infection.

How is it treated?

The most common treatment for a bacterial infection is an antibiotic to kill the invading organism. In case of a severe infection, such as a foot injury, your doctor may perform a procedure to clean the injured area and remove infected tissue.

You can reduce your risk of gum disease by brushing and flossing your teeth regularly. You can reduce your risk of a bladder infection by going to the bathroom regularly and making sure to empty your bladder.

Questions and answers

If I experience diabetic coma and no one is around to help me, will I eventually come out of it?

A comatose condition can result from dangerously high or low blood glucose. Whether consciousness is regained without assistance depends on many factors, including how high or low your blood glucose level is and how long it has been since you last ate or last received an insulin injection.

If you live alone or are by yourself for much of the day, recruit family members or friends to give you a call if you don't show up for work or to check on you periodically. It may seem like imposing, but these people are often happy to help, and they may even save your life.

My wife has episodes of hypoglycemia (severe low blood glucose). If she ever loses consciousness due to hypoglycemia, what should I do?

If she's in a coma because of hypoglycemia, the best immediate action is to give her a glucagon injection if you know how to do this. Because glucagon can cause vomiting, roll her to her side before giving the injection so she doesn't choke. If needed, call for emergency medical assistance.

If you find her at an earlier stage, when she may be confused but still alert, give her something that contains sugar to eat or drink to raise her blood glucose level. But never try to give food or drink to her if she's unconscious — she could choke. If she doesn't respond to the food or drink, give her a glucagon injection or call for immediate medical help.

Is the risk of death after a heart attack higher in people with diabetes than in people who don't have diabetes?

Yes. People with diabetes are more likely to have high blood pressure and high cholesterol, which increase damage to those arteries that supply oxygen to the heart (coronary arteries), causing a more severe attack. In addition, people with diabetes are less likely to experience typical symptoms of a heart attack, so they may not seek medical attention as quickly.

Can children with diabetes have heart attacks?

Not usually. Although people with type 1 diabetes usually develop the disease as children, they tend not to get heart disease until they reach adulthood.

How likely am I to already have eye damage by the time I'm diagnosed with diabetes?

Up to 30 percent of people with type 2 diabetes have eye damage (diabetic retinopathy) when they're first diagnosed. While initial eye damage may be minimal and not interfere with normal vision, it increases your risk of more serious eye disease. Because type 1 diabetes typically develops faster than type 2, people with type 1 diabetes are less likely to have retinopathy when first diagnosed. But the longer you have diabetes — whether it's type 1 or 2 — the higher your risk of retinopathy.

Part 2

Taking control

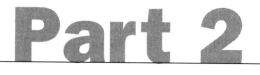

Chapter 3

Monitoring your blood glucose

C ontrol. That word comes up again and again, and for good reason. If you have diabetes, controlling your blood sugar (glucose) level is the single most important thing you can do to feel your best and prevent long-term complications.

But how do you achieve control? The cornerstones to controlling diabetes are:

- Monitoring your blood glucose
- Eating a healthy diet
- Staying active
- Maintaining a healthy weight
- Using medications appropriately, when necessary

This chapter focuses on the first of these five behaviors. Blood glucose monitoring is essential — it's the only way to know whether you're achieving your treatment goals.

If you've just been diagnosed with diabetes, or your treatment has changed, monitoring can seem overwhelming at first. You might feel angry, upset or fearful about having diabetes. You may be anxious about testing — afraid that it will take over your life, that it will be painful or disruptive. These feelings are normal. But as you learn how to measure your blood glucose and understand how regular testing can help you, you'll feel more comfortable with the procedure and more in control of your disease.

Know your goals

You want your blood glucose to stay within a desirable range — not too high or too low. This range is often referred to as your target range or your blood glucose goal. The normal range for a fasting blood glucose level is 70 to 100 milligrams of glucose per deciliter of blood (mg/dL). Ideally, that's the level at which you want to keep your blood glucose before meals. But that's not realistic for most people with diabetes. Instead, your focus may be on a range that's near normal.

Your doctor will help you determine your blood glucose goals. Because blood glucose naturally rises following a meal, your goal after meals will be different than before meals. Your goal before bed also may be different than during the day.

In determining your goals, your doctor takes into account several factors, including your age, whether you have any diabetes-related complications or other medical conditions, and how good you are at recognizing when your blood glucose is low. Recognizing symptoms of low blood glucose (hypoglycemia) is important because if your blood glucose drops too low, you may lose consciousness or have a seizure.

Below are typical goals for adults with diabetes.
- Before meals: 90 to 130 mg/dL
- About one to two hours after a meal: Under 180 mg/dL
- Before bedtime: 110 to 150 mg/dL

Your goals may differ, especially if you have complications, or you're pregnant, or you're older — so always follow the advice of your doctor.

When to test

How often you need to test your blood glucose and at what time of day depend on the type of diabetes you have and your treatment plan.

If you take insulin, you should test your blood glucose frequently, at least twice a day. Your doctor may advise testing three or four times a day or even more often.

Testing is commonly done before meals and at bedtime — in other words, when you haven't eaten for four or more hours. Your doctor may also advise you to test one to two hours after a meal. It's best to test your blood glucose just before your insulin injection.

A change in your regular routine may be another reason to test your blood glucose, especially if you have type 1 diabetes. This may include exercising more than normal, eating less than usual or traveling. Special circumstances, including pregnancy or illness, also may warrant increased testing.

If you have type 2 diabetes and you don't need insulin, test your blood glucose as often as necessary to make sure it's under control. For some people this may mean daily testing, while for others it might be twice a week. In general, if you're able to control your blood glucose with diet and exercise, and without using medication, you don't need to test your blood glucose as often.

Your doctor or a diabetes educator (explained on page 154) can help you determine a monitoring schedule that's right for you.

Tools you need

Testing your blood glucose is a quick and easy process that generally takes less than two minutes. You'll need these tools:

Lancet and lancing device. A lancet is a small needle that pricks the skin on your finger so that you can draw a drop of blood. A lancing device holds the lancet. Spring-loaded lancing devices are generally less painful than other types. Because people differ in skin thickness, lancets can usually be set for different prick depths using a dial.

Test strips. Test strips are chemically treated — you place blood from your finger (or another site) on these strips. If you have a newer blood glucose monitor, you'll insert the strip into the monitor first, before drawing blood. With older models the strip is inserted after blood is applied to it.

Blood glucose meter. A blood glucose meter, also called a blood glucose monitor, is a small, computerized device that measures and displays your blood glucose level.

Choosing the right meter

Blood glucose meters come in many forms with a variety of features. So how do you know which device is right for you? Your diabetes educator or doctor may recommend a meter or help you select one. Keep in mind that some health plans require their participants to use a specific meter.

When choosing a meter, consider these factors:

Cost. Most insurance plans and Medicare cover the cost of a blood glucose meter and test strips (after you pay your deductible and any coinsurance). Find out what your insurance covers before you buy. Some plans limit the total number of test strips allowed. Meters vary widely in price, so shop around before you buy.

The test strips are the most expensive part of monitoring because they're used so often. Strips that are individually packaged tend to cost more, but you might not use all the strips in a container before the expiration date or within the required number of days after opening the container. Figure out which type of strip is most cost-effective for you.

Ease of use and maintenance. Some meters are easier to use than others. Are the meter and strips comfortable to hold? Can you easily see the numbers on the screen? How easy is it to get blood onto the strips? Does it require a small or large drop of blood? Find out how the meter is calibrated, that is, how it's set or coded for the test strips. How often will you have to recalibrate the meter? How often do you have to change the batteries?

Special features. Ask about the features to see what meets your specific needs. For example, some meters are large with strips that are easier to handle. Some are compact and easier to carry. People with impaired vision can buy a meter with a large screen or a "talking" meter that announces the results. For children there are colorful meters that give a quick reading.

Also consider how the meter stores and retrieves information. Some can track all the information you'd normally write in a log, such as the time and date of a test, the result and trends over time. You can even download this information into a computer to chart your diabetes management.

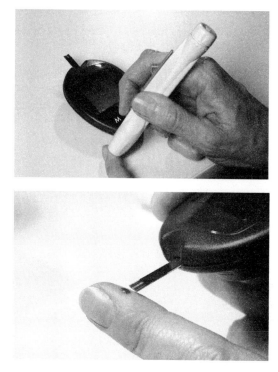

Puncture your fingertip
Place the tip covering the lancet on the side of your fingertip. Because the flat side of your fingertip is more sensitive, you may want to prick the side of your finger, as shown. Press the button to discharge the lancet.

Touch test strip to blood
Hold your hand down to encourage a drop of blood to form. If the blood doesn't come out easily, gently squeeze the end of your finger. Avoid touching your skin with the test strip. Instead, touch the drop of blood.

Performing the test

Follow the instructions that come with your glucose meter. But in general, here's the procedure:

- Before pricking your finger, wash your hands with soap and warm water. Dry them well.
- Remove a test strip from the container and replace the cap immediately to prevent damage to the strips.
- Insert the test strip into the meter.
- With a lancet, stick the side of your finger, not the tip, so that you won't have sore spots on the part of your finger you use the most.
- When you have a drop of blood, touch the test strip to the blood (avoid touching your skin with the test strip) and wait for a reading. Within a few seconds, the meter displays your blood glucose level on a screen.

Your fingertips have a lot of nerve endings, so rotate the sites where you stick your fingers. If you have a newer glucose meter, you'll have the option to test your blood glucose from other sites. But check with your doctor or diabetes educator first to find out if alternative site testing is appropriate in your case.

Alternative site testing

Newer glucose meters offer what's called alternative site testing. That means you can test your blood from sites other than the fingertip — such as the palm, forearm, upper arm and thigh. But the Food and Drug Administration (FDA) points out that blood from your fingertips shows changes in glucose levels (after a meal or exercise, for example) more quickly than blood from other sites. In other words, results from other sites may not always be as accurate.

Use blood from your fingertip rather than other sites if:
- You think your blood glucose is low
- Your blood glucose is rapidly changing because of food or medication
- You've just finished exercising
- You suspect that the results from the alternative site are unreliable

When using an alternative site, you'll need to massage the puncture site to stimulate the flow of blood before you use the lancing device. Check the instructions that come with the glucose meter to see which sites the FDA approved for the product you're using. Ask your doctor or diabetes educator if it's acceptable to use sites other than your fingertip.

Are you getting quality results?

Blood glucose meters are generally accurate and precise. Human error rather than a nonfunctioning machine is more likely to produce an inaccurate reading. To ensure accurate results, follow each step carefully.

To check your meter and your testing skill, take your meter along when you visit your doctor or have an appointment for lab work. Your doctor or diabetes educator can have you check your blood glucose at the same time that blood is drawn for lab tests. That way you can compare the reading you get with the lab results. Your meter results shouldn't be off by more than 15 percent.

In addition, once a week, do a quality control test of your equipment and technique. It's also a good idea to do the test when you start a new container of test strips or you calibrate the meter or change the batteries.

To do a quality control test, follow your normal blood-testing procedure, but use a liquid control solution instead of blood. These solutions are available at most drugstores and pharmacies and come in three ranges: high, normal or low. Ask your diabetes educator which solution to use.

If your results aren't acceptable

Acceptable values for the control test are listed in the insert that comes with the control solution or with the test strips. If the results of your control test don't fall within the acceptable range, do the following:

Check the strips. Throw out damaged or outdated strips.

Check the control solution. Check the expiration date and use fresh solution, if necessary.

Check the meter. Make sure the strip guide and the test window (if it has one) are clean. Follow the manufacturer's instructions for cleaning. Replace batteries if they're weak.

Check the calibration (measurement scale) of the meter. Some meters are calibrated in the factory and have a check strip or paddle that can be inserted to verify the calibration. Others are calibrated to each container of strips. Make sure you're using strips that have been calibrated for your meter. Be sure the code number in the meter matches the code number on the strip container.

Other problems that can lead to an inaccurate reading include:
- Not enough blood applied to the test strip
- More blood added to the test strip after the first drop was applied
- Alcohol, dirt or other substances on your finger or alternative site
- A meter that's not at room temperature
- A damaged meter

After you've corrected potential problems, repeat the control test. If the results are still unacceptable, talk to your diabetes educator or call the meter manufacturer for help.

Recording your results

More than just providing an immediate measurement of your blood glucose, monitoring can help you assess your progress in managing your diabetes. Each time you perform a blood test, log your results. This information helps you see how food, physical activity, medication and other factors affect your blood glucose. As patterns occur, you can begin to understand how your daily activities affect your blood glucose level. This puts you in a better position to manage your diabetes day by day and even hour by hour.

Your life is not the same from one day to the next. Some days you exercise more or eat less. Maybe you're sick or you're having trouble at work or home. These changes affect your blood glucose level. By keeping an accurate record of day-to-day events and your blood glucose levels, you'll find problem areas and will be better able to maintain good control.

With the information you gain, you can anticipate problems before they occur. You can plan ahead for changes in your routine that you know will affect your blood glucose, such as traveling, eating out or working harder than usual.

What to track

Your diabetes educator or doctor may have given you a record book for recording your test results. If not, you can use any type of notebook. You also can keep your results on a computer. Many software programs are available for recording and tracking blood glucose levels — ask your health care team what they recommend.

Every time you check your blood glucose, record:
- The date and time
- The test result
- The type and dosage of medication you're taking

Also include information that can help explain a change from your normal blood glucose level, such as:
- A change in your diet (for example, having a birthday dinner, eating at a restaurant or eating more than usual)
- A change in your exercise or activity level
- Unusual excitement or stress

Magic numbers

When you're testing and recording your blood glucose frequently, it's easy to get caught up in a numbers game. The right numbers equal success, while the wrong numbers represent failure. You may end up feeling upset, confused, angry, frustrated or discouraged about your blood glucose results.

It's also easy to become obsessive about testing and test results. If you're already a perfectionist or on the obsessive side, you can go overboard with all the numbers and record keeping involved in monitoring your blood glucose.

There's nothing magical about these numbers. They're a tool to help you track how well your treatment plan is working. Your results can indicate if you need to make changes in your treatment. No matter how well you're doing with your plan or how hard you try, your blood glucose readings won't be perfect every time. Sometimes "bad" readings happen for no apparent reason.

- An illness
- An insulin reaction

Take your record book with you when you see your doctor, diabetes educator or dietitian. He or she can help you interpret the results. Based on the information that you track, your doctor may recommend changes in your medication and discuss your diet, level of physical activity and other lifestyle issues. The more complete your records are, the more useful they'll be.

Factors that affect blood glucose

The amount of glucose in your blood continuously varies. That's because many factors affect how your body metabolizes food into glucose and how it uses this glucose. Self-monitoring helps you learn what makes your blood glucose level rise and fall so that you can make adjustments in your treatment. It also can help you understand why your blood glucose level may be different from day to day or hour to hour.

Food

Food raises your blood glucose level. One to two hours after a meal, your blood glucose is at its highest level. Then it starts to fall. What you eat, how much you eat and at what time you eat all affect your blood glucose level.

Strive for consistency from day to day in the time you eat and the amount of food you eat. By controlling when and how much you eat, you control the times your blood glucose is higher, such as after meals. You also control how high your blood glucose rises. If you eat too much, your blood glucose will be higher than usual. Too little food may result in lower than usual blood glucose. If you take insulin, this could put you at risk of hypoglycemia (see page 22).

It's also important to understand that different foods have a different effect on your blood glucose. Food is made up of carbohydrates, protein and fat. All three increase blood glucose, but carbohydrates have the most noticeable effect. Even within the carbohydrates group, different types have varying effects on blood glucose.

Your liver

As mentioned in Chapter 1, glucose is stored in your liver in a form called glycogen. Your liver also makes new glucose from other substances, such as protein and fat. When your blood glucose level falls, your liver breaks down glycogen and releases it into your bloodstream. This generally happens when you haven't eaten for a while. The continuous process of storing and releasing glucose causes natural variations in everyone's blood glucose levels, but it's more pronounced when you have diabetes.

Exercise and physical activity

Typically, exercise and physical activity lower your blood glucose level. With help from insulin, exercise and physical activity promote the transfer of glucose from your blood to your cells, where the glucose is used for energy. The more you exercise, the more glucose you use and the faster it's transported to cells, lowering the amount of glucose in your blood. Exercise also reduces insulin resistance, making your cells more responsive to insulin, so insulin works more efficiently.

Although fairly uncommon, sometimes exercise has the opposite effect — it raises your blood glucose. This usually happens if your blood glucose is very high to begin with — typically more than 300 mg/dL. Until you know how your body responds to exercise, test your blood glucose before and after exercising and again several hours later. (See "Exercise and blood glucose monitoring," page 99.)

Medications

Insulin and oral diabetes medications lower your blood glucose level. The time of day you take your medication and how much you take affect how much your blood glucose level drops. If your medication is causing your blood glucose to drop too much, or not enough, your doctor may need to make adjustments to your dosage.

Medications taken for other conditions also can affect blood glucose. Whenever you're prescribed a new medication for another health condition, remind your doctor that you have diabetes and ask if the medication may alter your blood glucose level. By being aware of its effects and following simple precautions, such as increased glucose monitoring, you may keep it from causing significant changes in your blood glucose levels. If the drug does make it harder for you to control your blood glucose, talk with your doctor.

Illness

The physical stress of a cold, influenza or other illness, especially a bacterial infection, causes your body to produce hormones that increase blood glucose. Injury or a major health problem such as a heart attack also can increase blood glucose. The additional glucose helps to promote healing. But in people with diabetes, more glucose can be a problem. When you're sick it's important to monitor your blood glucose frequently.

Alcohol

Alcohol prevents your liver from releasing glucose and can increase the risk of your blood glucose falling too low. If you take insulin or oral diabetes medications, you risk experiencing low blood glucose (hypoglycemia) when you drink alcohol — even as little as 2 ounces. If you choose to drink alcohol, drink only in moderation.

To prevent your blood glucose from dropping too low, never drink on an empty stomach or if your blood glucose is already low. (See "Is it OK to drink alcohol?" page 71.)

Less commonly, alcohol can do the opposite — cause your blood glucose to rise. This could happen, for example, with the sugary sodas or juices used in mixed drinks. Monitor your blood glucose before and after drinking alcohol to see how your body responds to its use.

Overcoming barriers to testing

Despite its advantages, many people with diabetes don't test their blood glucose as often as they should — or at all. Reasons and suggested solutions include:

Cost. Many diabetes supply companies offer low-cost supplies. In addition, many diabetes drug companies have patient assistance programs. If cost is a factor for you, talk with your doctor or diabetes educator and ask if there's a local or nationwide program that can help defray your expenses.

Limited access to health care. If getting to a medical center is a problem, check with your local, county or state health department about outreach health care services.

Lack of information and misperceptions. Some people are simply unaware of the benefits of blood glucose monitoring and believe there is nothing they can do to improve their disease. One of the best weapons in managing diabetes is education. Learn as much as you can about your disease.

Fear. If you fear the discomfort of pricking your finger, keep in mind that newer lancets are less painful.

Lifestyle issues. Even with a hectic or unconventional work schedule, you can find ways to build monitoring into your daily routine. Your doctor or diabetes educator can help with this.

Privacy issues. Testing is quick and monitors are portable. You may be able to find a private place, such as a bathroom, to do your tests. But if you have to check your blood glucose in public, remember millions of people do it every day.

When test results signal a problem

Watch for patterns that show your blood glucose readings are persistently above or below your goals. This might indicate that your medication needs to be adjusted or, if you're not taking medication, that your diet and exercise efforts aren't enough to control your blood glucose. Persistent high or low blood glucose readings put you at risk of complications of diabetes.

Having high or low blood glucose once in a while — especially if you can identify the reason — isn't cause for alarm. However, frequent, unexplained high or low blood glucose readings need medical attention.

Call your doctor if:

- Your blood glucose is persistently higher than 300 mg/dL
- Your blood glucose readings are persistently above or below your goals
- Your blood glucose is greater than 250 mg/dL for more than 24 hours during an illness
- You frequently have low blood glucose (hypoglycemia)

Advances in blood glucose monitoring

Blood testing tools are always changing. Less invasive and faster devices are now on the market or in development, but that doesn't mean they're equally accurate in their results.

The FDA tests and approves all new products that help monitor your blood glucose. Some blood glucose meters require a prescription and some are approved for testing other sites, in addition to your fingertip. New blood glucose meters and features highlighted by their marketers include, for example:

- A disposable glucose meter with 100 preloaded test strips
- A compact meter (3 inches by 1.5 inches) that gives results in about seven seconds and has reminder alarms when it's time to test
- A meter that requires no coding (calibration) and has symbols that indicate when to apply the blood sample, whether the meter is too hot or too cold to use, or if the battery is low

Other monitoring devices

A monitoring device that's worn like a wristwatch doesn't puncture your skin to measure glucose. Instead, small electrical currents draw tiny amounts of fluid from the skin toward a special sensor pad to measure glucose. It stores readings so that you can track patterns and trends. An alarm sounds if your blood glucose level becomes too low or too high. Finger-stick tests are still required when you use this system, although not as frequently.

A monitoring system being developed but not yet available involves wearing a patch on your arm for several minutes. The patch draws glucose from fluid in your skin, and results are read with a portable meter.

Another system under development uses light to determine the blood glucose level in the fluid between your cells (interstitial fluid). The light shines through your skin, and the amount of light absorbed would be an indicator of glucose level.

Watch for new developments, but always discuss what's best for your needs with your doctor or diabetes educator before buying a new blood glucose monitoring device.

Questions and answers

Should I be testing glucose in my urine? Is that done anymore?
In the past, the only practical way for people with diabetes to monitor their glucose was by testing glucose in their urine. But urine glucose tests aren't as accurate as blood glucose tests. They provide only a rough estimate of your blood glucose level. And urine tests don't detect glucose levels lower than 180 mg/dL, so they can't detect low blood glucose. (See "Urine testing at home," page 162.)

Does stress affect blood glucose?
Stress can affect blood glucose in two ways. When you're under a lot of stress, it's easy to abandon your usual routine. You may exercise less, eat less healthy foods and not test your blood glucose as often. As a result stress indirectly causes your blood glucose to rise.

Occasionally, stress can have a direct effect on your blood glucose level. Physical and psychological stress may cause your body to produce hormones that prevent insulin from working properly, increasing blood glucose levels. This tends to be more common in people with type 2 diabetes.

To find out how you react to stress, log your stress level on a scale of 1 to 10 every time you log your blood glucose level. After a couple of weeks, look for a pattern. Do high blood glucose levels often occur with high stress levels and low blood glucose levels with low stress? If so, stress may be affecting your blood glucose control — discuss this with your doctor or diabetes educator.

Can heat affect my blood glucose level?

Heat doesn't have a direct effect on your blood glucose, but it might lead you to change your daily routine. On hot days, for example, you may eat less than usual or exert yourself more. These changes could lower your blood glucose. Whenever your daily routine changes, test your glucose more often.

Sunburn also can affect blood glucose control. A severe sunburn is stressful to the body, and like other physical stresses, it can raise your blood glucose. Use a good sunscreen and wear sunglasses and a hat when you're out in the sun.

What's the difference between whole blood glucose levels and plasma blood glucose levels?

Home glucose meters use whole blood to measure glucose levels. But when blood is drawn at your medical appointment and sent to a lab, the red blood cells are removed, leaving only plasma, before glucose is measured. Because of this difference, results from labs and home monitors aren't exactly the same.

Plasma tests tend to be more accurate, and the results are 10 percent to 15 percent higher than whole blood test results. But most home meters (especially new ones) are calibrated to give a plasma test result, even though they use whole blood for the test. Your home monitor's results are considered accurate if they fall within 15 percent of the lab test result.

My doctor told me that I have prediabetes. I'm scheduled to have heart bypass surgery soon and was told that I might need insulin to control my blood glucose when I'm in the hospital. Why would I need insulin if I don't have diabetes?

Studies show that people with high blood glucose (hyperglycemia) often do better when hospitalized if their blood glucose is carefully monitored and controlled, even if they don't have a diagnosis of diabetes. Some hospital patients with hyperglycemia may require insulin, depending on their glucose levels. If your glucose gets out of control while you're in the hospital, it could increase your risk of complications such as infections, organ failure and even death. Most people with prediabetes go on to develop type 2 diabetes unless they change their lifestyle so that they eat healthy, increase their physical activity and achieve a healthy weight.

Do I need to adjust my monitoring routine when I'm traveling?

You can still get out and see the world if you have diabetes. It just takes a little more planning. When you travel, bring at least twice the medication and testing supplies as you think you'll need.

Because stress, time changes, and changes in your eating and sleeping schedule can affect your blood glucose level, it's a good idea to test it more frequently than normal. If you're flying, especially for a long period, test your blood glucose level as soon as possible after landing. Jet lag can make you tired or fatigued, making it more difficult to tell if you have low or high blood glucose.

Chapter 4

Developing a healthy-eating plan

D o the words *healthy eating* produce a twinge of fear? Some people may think, "Oh no, I'll never get to eat my favorite treats again!" But healthy eating isn't about deprivation or denial. It means enjoying great nutrition as well as great taste. Healthy eating can mean updating your routine fare with delicious foods that you haven't tried before and experimenting with recipes to make them tasty as well as nutritious.

A healthy diet is key to a healthy life, especially if you have diabetes or if you're at risk.

There is no diabetes diet

Contrary to popular myth, having diabetes doesn't mean that you have to start eating special foods or follow a complicated diet plan. For most people, having diabetes simply translates into eating a variety of foods in moderate amounts and sticking to regular mealtimes.

This means choosing a diet that emphasizes vegetables, fruits and whole grains — and smaller servings of lean or low-fat animal foods, such as lean cuts of meat and low-fat dairy products. This kind of diet is naturally nutrient-rich and low in fat and calories. It's the same eating plan that all Americans should follow.

Depending on your blood sugar (glucose) level, whether you need to lose weight and whether you have other health problems, you may need to tailor your diet somewhat to meet your personal needs. But even though the details may differ, the basics remain the same. Each day you want to eat a variety of foods to achieve the right balance of three key nutrients: carbohydrates, protein and fats.

Target 3 key nutrients: Eat a variety of foods

Nutrient	Aim for	Number of grams*
Carbohydrates	45% to 65% of daily calories	225 to 325 grams (g)
Protein	15% to 20% of daily calories	75 to 100 g (1 ounce of protein food contains about 7 g)
Fats	20% to 35% of daily calories, but less than 10% from saturated fat and less than 1% from trans fat	44 to 78 g (less than 22 g of saturated fat and less than 2 g of trans fat)

*This is based on a 2,000-calorie diet for adults. Recommendations vary if you're on a higher or lower calorie diet or if you have certain health conditions, so check with your doctor for advice.

Based on the Dietary Guidelines for Americans, 2005

Carbohydrates: The foundation

Carbohydrates are your body's main energy source. During digestion all carbohydrates, except fiber, break down into blood glucose. Your brain, for example, uses glucose as its primary source of fuel. The three main categories of carbohydrates are explained in the box on the next page.

Main types of carbohydrates	
Category	**Includes**
Sugars (also called simple carbohydrates)	*Natural sugars:* Found in foods such as fruits, milk, milk products (cheese and yogurt, for example) — when choosing dairy products, focus on low-fat and fat-free. *Added sugars:* Added to foods such as desserts and candy; includes table sugar, honey, jelly, syrups and other processed sweets — generally, these foods are high in calories with little nutritional value.
Starches (also called complex carbohydrates)	*Legumes:* Beans, peas and lentils, for example *Starchy vegetables:* Potatoes, squash, corn and others *Grains:* Wheat, oats, barley, rice and rye — for heart health and other benefits, focus on whole grains, found in products such as whole-grain bread, whole-wheat cereal, oatmeal, brown rice, wild rice and whole-wheat pasta.
Fiber	*Soluble fiber:* Sources such as unprocessed (unrefined) oats, barley, and many fruits and vegetables — eating large amounts of soluble fiber may slow the rise of blood glucose and help lower cholesterol. *Insoluble fiber:* Sources such as wheat bran and skins of fruits and vegetables — insoluble fiber adds bulk and aids digestion.

Combining your carbs

About half of your daily calories should come from carbohydrates. The number of servings depends on your calorie needs — ask your doctor or dietitian what's best for you. General recommendations for all adults, based on the 2005 Dietary Guidelines for Americans, include:

- 6 ounces of grains — at least half from whole grains (for example, 1 ounce equals one slice of whole-grain bread or five low-fat whole-wheat crackers or $^1/_2$ cup of brown rice)
- At least $2^1/_2$ cups of vegetables (include a variety)
- At least 2 cups of fruit (include a variety)
- 3 cups of fat-free or low-fat milk products

To help control your glucose level, eat about the same amount of carbohydrates each day, spaced throughout the day. If you eat more or fewer carbohydrates than usual at a meal or from day to day, you may cause your glucose level to vary.

The scoop on sugar

For decades, people with diabetes were told to avoid sugar. And this is still a common misconception when people first learn they have diabetes — that they'll have to give up sweets for good. But things have changed. Here's why.

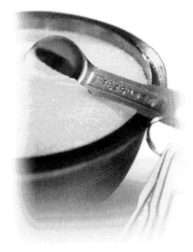

For years, medical professionals assumed that honey, candy and other sweets would raise your blood glucose faster and higher than fruits, vegetables or foods containing complex carbohydrates. But many studies have shown this isn't true, provided that they're eaten with your meal and counted as a carbohydrate source.

It's still best to eat sugar in moderation. Sweet foods, such as candy, cookies or soda pop, have little nutritional value and are often high in fat and calories. You receive empty calories without the nutrients that your body needs to function. In addition, those extra calories can lead to weight gain.

After eating a sugary food, test your blood glucose and observe its effect, which may differ with different types of sweets. You can use sugar-free products that contain artificial sweeteners, but keep in mind that some of these sugar-free foods may still be high in total calories.

Special diets

If you have another health condition in addition to diabetes, such as high blood pressure or kidney disease, your doctor may recommend that you modify your diet to help that condition, too.

Low sodium diet

Lowering the amount of sodium you eat helps prevent too much sodium from building up in your body. This may help reduce blood pressure and the tendency to retain fluids. Limiting sodium may also help your heart work more efficiently.

Some sodium is found naturally in fresh and unprocessed foods, so it's impossible — and unnecessary — to go on a "no sodium diet." Most of the sodium that people consume comes from salt (sodium chloride) and sodium preservatives added to many processed foods. A low sodium diet omits or limits processed foods that are especially high in salt, such as salted soups, salted canned vegetables, salty or smoked meats, bottled sauces (soy sauce, ketchup, mustard), processed cheeses, salted snacks, pickles, olives and frozen convenience foods.

The 2005 Dietary Guidelines for Americans recommends that people with high blood pressure, blacks, and middle-aged and older adults limit their sodium intake to 1,500 miligrams (mg) a day.

Low protein, low potassium diet

When you have kidney disease, your kidneys have problems performing their normal functions, including regulating the amount of minerals such as sodium and potassium in your body, and removing waste products that are produced when protein is broken down.

If your kidneys aren't functioning properly, these minerals and protein byproducts can build up in your blood and tissues, and you may need to tailor your diet to limit their consumption. A dietitian can help you learn what foods to eat and which to limit or avoid.

Protein: The building block

Your body uses protein for the development and maintenance of your muscles and organs. Foods high in protein include meat, poultry, eggs, cheese, fish, legumes and peanut butter. If you eat more protein than you need — which many people do — your body stores the extra calories from protein as fat.

For most people, a healthy diet includes 15 percent to 20 percent of their daily calories from protein — the amount of protein depends on your calorie needs. For example, if you're on a 2,000-calorie diet, that means 75 to 100 grams (g) of protein a day, such as:

- 3 to 5 ounces of poultry, fish or lean meat (20 to 35 g of protein)
- Three servings of fat-free milk products (about 24 g of protein)
- Common starches and vegetables for the remainder

Select proteins that are lower in fat, such as fish, poultry without skin, lean meats, and low-fat or fat-free cheese. Whether or not you're a vegetarian, plant sources of protein, such as legumes (beans, dried peas and lentils) and products made from soy (miso, seitan, tempeh, tofu, soy milk and soy cheese) can replace meat and dairy products. These foods are also low in fat and cholesterol. Never heard of some of these foods? Consider this an opportunity to try something new.

Fats: The calorie heavyweights

Fats are the most concentrated source of food energy, providing lots of calories but little nutrition. Yet a small amount of certain fats are essential to the life and function of your cells. It's when you eat too much fat — and the wrong kinds — that health problems occur.

Not all fats are created equal as described in the box on the next page. Still, all fats are high in calories, so limit total fat consumption. (See "Fats" in the box page 58.)

Cutting down on fat
To limit the amount of fat you eat and help control blood glucose and blood fats, follow these tips:

- Choose fat-free or low-fat products.
- Use canola or olive oil (in small amounts) for cooking and salads.
- Buy lean cuts of meat and trim off the excess fat.
- Marinate meats and use herbs and spices to keep them tender, moist and give them flavor.
- Remove the skin from poultry before cooking.
- Avoid fried foods. Instead, bake, steam, grill, broil or roast meat and vegetables.
- Season vegetables with lemon, lime or herbs rather than butter or oil.
- Replace some of the shortening in baked goods with applesauce or prune purée.

Fats: The good and the bad

As you read labels, look for products that contain monounsaturated fats with little or no saturated and trans fats. Remember that all fats are high in calories.

Monounsaturated fats ("good fats") help lower total and "bad" LDL (low-density lipoprotein) cholesterol and are more resistant to oxidation. Oxidation promotes the absorption of fats and cholesterol into artery walls, speeding the buildup of artery-clogging plaques. *Found mainly in:* Olive, canola and peanut oils, as well as most nuts and avocados.

Polyunsaturated fats help lower total and "bad" LDL cholesterol, but these fats also seem susceptible to the harmful process of oxidation. *Found mainly in:* Vegetable oils such as safflower, corn, sunflower, soy and cottonseed.

Saturated fats raise total and "bad" LDL cholesterol, increasing your risk of heart disease. *Found mainly in:* Red meats, most whole-fat dairy products (including butter), egg yolks, chocolate (cocoa butter), as well as coconut, palm and other tropical oils.

Trans fats, also called hydrogenated or partially hydrogenated vegetable oil, raise "bad" LDL cholesterol, increasing your risk of heart disease. *Found mainly in:* Stick margarine and shortening and the products made from them — cookies, pastry, other baked goods, most crackers, candies, snack foods and french fries.

Get your omega-3s

Eating fish that are rich in omega-3 fatty acids can help protect against coronary artery disease. Fish high in omega-3 fats include anchovies, bass (striped, sea and freshwater), bluefish, herring, salmon, sardines, trout (rainbow and lake) and tuna (especially white, albacore and bluefin), among others.* Eating at least two, 3-ounce servings of these types of fish every week is recommended as part of a heart-healthy diet.

*The Food and Drug Administration advises pregnant women, nursing mothers and children not to eat king mackerel, shark, swordfish or tilefish because these types of fish have higher amounts of mercury.

Planning your meals

A meal plan is simply an eating guide with two key points:
1. It helps establish a routine for eating meals and snacks at regular times every day.
2. It guides you in choosing the healthiest foods in the right amounts at each meal.

When you're first diagnosed with diabetes, talk with your doctor about your eating habits. Eating at irregular times, overeating or making poor food choices often contributes to high blood glucose. Your doctor can provide you with a variety of tips to help you change your eating habits to achieve better glucose control.

Some people may need to follow a more deliberate plan, eating only the recommended number of servings from each food group every day, based on their individual calorie needs. Depending on your blood glucose control, your doctor may want you to meet with a dietitian to help you improve your eating habits and better manage your diabetes.

Working with a dietitian

Understanding what foods to eat, how much to eat and how your food choices affect your blood glucose level can be a complex task. A registered dietitian can help you make sense of all this information and put together a plan that's easy to follow and that fits your health goals, food tastes, family or cultural traditions, and lifestyle.

At the first meeting, the dietitian typically asks about your weight history and your eating habits — what you like to eat, how much you eat, as well as when and what time of day you have meals and snacks. You'll usually discuss your diabetes treatment goals, what medications you take, any special health considerations, calorie needs, whether you're trying to lose weight, physical activity level and your work schedule.

Together you and your dietitian will figure out what's practical and achievable for you. And you'll both decide on the best meal-planning tool to help you control your diabetes. The most common tools for planning meals are carbohydrate counting and exchange lists.

Medicare covers some medical nutrition therapy

If you have diabetes and you're covered under Medicare Part B, you may be eligible for medical nutrition therapy services if your doctor prescribes them. This means that, after you've paid your deductible for Part B services, Medicare pays 80 percent of the cost of a limited number of hours of nutrition counseling by a registered dietitian. Ask your doctor for more information.

Carb counting as a meal-planning tool

Some people with diabetes — especially those who take diabetes medications or insulin — use carbohydrate counting as a meal-planning tool. They count the amount of carbohydrates in each meal or snack and adjust their insulin dose to the amount of carbohydrates. This helps keep their blood glucose from going too high or too low throughout the day.

The amount of protein and fat in the meal generally isn't taken into consideration when determining the insulin dose. However, carbohydrate counting doesn't mean that you can go overboard on foods that are low in carbohydrates or that don't contain any carbohydrates, such as meat and fats. Remember, too many calories and too much fat and cholesterol over the long term increases your risk of weight gain, heart disease, stroke and other diseases.

Is the glycemic index a good meal-planning tool?

The glycemic index (GI) ranks carbohydrate-containing foods based on their effect on blood glucose levels. High-index foods are associated with greater increases in blood glucose than low-index foods. But low-index foods aren't necessarily healthier. Foods that are high in fat tend to have lower GI values than do some healthy foods.

Using the GI for meal planning is a fairly complicated process. Many factors affect the GI value of a specific food, such as how the food was prepared and what you eat with it. Also, the GI value for some foods isn't known.

Another meal-planning tool is the glycemic load, which multiplies the GI of a food by the amount of total carbohydrates in a serving. For example, eating small amounts of a food with a high GI may have less impact on blood glucose.

Talk with a registered dietitian if you have questions. Currently there isn't enough evidence of benefits to recommend using GI diets as your main strategy in meal planning.

Be consistent. Large variations in carbohydrate intake throughout the day — skipping meals, then eating huge meals — can cause blood glucose levels to go too high or too low.

Don't confuse carb counting with fad diets, such as low-carb (low-carbohydrate) diets. In addition, the terms *net carbohydrates* or *net carbs* on product labels can be misleading. These marketing terms aren't approved by the Food and Drug Administration (FDA), so you may not accurately count your carbohydrates if you use the net carb number on the label. And if you're on insulin, you could underestimate how much you need.

If you're counting carbohydrates, work with your dietitian to learn how to do it properly to meet your specific needs.

Exchange lists

Your dietitian may recommend using a booklet that lists foods by food group and serving size, called an exchange list. In the exchange system, foods are grouped into these categories:

- Starches
- Nonstarchy vegetables
- Fruits
- Meat and meat substitutes
- Milk and milk products
- Fats
- Sweets, desserts and other carbohydrates

You can exchange or trade foods within a group because they have about the same amount of carbohydrates, protein, fat and calories — so each exchange has about the same effect on your blood glucose. An exchange is basically one serving within a group. One starch exchange, for instance, might be half of a medium baked potato (3 ounces) or $1/3$ cup of baked beans or $1/2$ cup of corn.

Another list in the exchange system is called *free foods*. You can include some of these foods in your diabetes meal plan as often as you'd like — others you can enjoy in moderation. A free food means a food or drink that has fewer than 20 calories or no more than 5 grams of carbohydrates per serving. If you're overweight, your dietitian may caution you that foods with 5 grams or less of carbohydrates aren't "free" if they have a lot of calories.

Calculating exchanges for recipes

Your meal plan looks great, but there's one small problem: Where do your favorite recipes fit in? They're not on the food lists.

By following the steps below, you can figure out the exchange values for many of your favorite recipes and the number of exchanges each serving of a recipe provides.

1. List all the ingredients in a recipe and their amounts.
2. For each ingredient, write down the number of exchanges it provides. You'll probably have to consult a list of exchange values of commonly used ingredients. You can find this in many diabetic cookbooks or ask your dietitian for one.
3. Total each exchange group.
4. Divide the total number of exchanges for each group by the number of servings in the recipe and round off to the nearest $1/2$ exchange (round up for amounts greater than $1/2$ exchange).

A dietitian can help you use an exchange list to figure out your daily meal plan. He or she will recommend a certain number of servings from each food group based on your individual needs.

Not everyone with diabetes needs to use an exchange list, but many people with type 1 or type 2 diabetes find it helpful.

Consistency is key

If you're consistent in your eating habits, it'll help control your blood glucose levels. Every day try to eat:

- At about the same time
- The same number of meals and about the same amount of food

Stick to your meal plan. This ensures that you'll eat about the same percentages of carbohydrates, protein and fats every day. It's more difficult to control your blood glucose if you eat a big lunch one day and a small one the next. And the more you vary the amount of carbohydrates that you eat, the harder it is to control your blood glucose.

Eating at regularly spaced intervals — meals and planned snacks spaced four to five hours apart — reduces large variations in blood glucose and also allows for adequate digestion and metabolism of food.

Watch your serving sizes

Whether you count carbs or use exchange lists, pay close attention to serving sizes. With the trend toward supersizing, mega-buffets and huge portions in restaurants, you may not have an accurate idea of what a regular serving size is. Both of these meal-planning tools include guidelines for serving sizes. Use them — don't try to estimate.

At first, the serving sizes may seem small. Using exchange lists, 3 cups of popcorn (low-fat microwave or popped with no fat added) is one serving. This amount may hardly make a dent in the large bucket you're used to getting at the movies. But with better meal and snack planning, smaller servings of some foods allow you to enjoy a greater variety and amount of other foods. And you'll have better glucose control.

Sizing up a serving using exchange lists

Here are a few examples of what counts as one serving when you use exchange lists. Your meal plan may recommend several servings from each food group for every meal.

Food	Examples of one serving
Starches and grains	1 slice whole-wheat bread $1/4$ whole-grain bagel (1 ounce) $1/3$ cup whole-grain pasta or brown rice $3/4$ cup dry or $1/2$ cup cooked cereal $1/2$ baked potato, medium size (3 ounces)
Fruits and vegetables	$1/2$ cup 100 percent orange or apple juice 1 small apple or small banana (4 ounces each) $1/2$ cup fresh fruit 1 cup raw or $1/2$ cup cooked vegetables
Milk and milk products	1 cup low-fat or fat-free milk $2/3$ cup (6 ounces) plain fat-free yogurt
Meat and meat substitutes	1 ounce lean meat, fish or skinless poultry $1/4$ cup low-fat or fat-free cottage cheese* $1/2$ cup cooked beans or dried peas*

*This has as much protein as 1 ounce of meat.

Based on the American Diabetes Association and American Dietetic Association *Exchange Lists for Meal Planning*, 2003

How to estimate portions

Remember these visual cues to help you estimate how much food you're eating:

- $1/2$ cup = small ice-cream scoop or light bulb
- 1 teaspoon = tip of your thumb
- 1 tablespoon = entire thumb
- 1 cup = your fist
- 3 ounces (3 exchanges) meat, fish or chicken = deck of cards

Keep motivated

Sticking to a healthy-eating plan is one of the most challenging aspects of living with diabetes. The key is to find ways to keep motivated and overcome potential hurdles.

Financial concerns. Buying lots of fresh fruits and vegetables can be expensive. But keep in mind that you're probably buying fewer less nutritious foods, such as chips and sweets, which also can be costly. You can also save money if you buy less meat.

Cultural barriers. Food is an expression of culture. But all cuisine can be prepared in healthier ways. You can find cookbooks for people with diabetes that focus on foods from different cultures, with plenty of ideas for making recipes healthier.

Family and social situations. Sometimes family members and friends may not understand why you're making changes to your meals — and theirs. Discuss your diabetes treatment goals and ask them for their support. The changes you're making will help keep you and your family healthy. If family and friends seem offended if you say no to their special dishes, enlist their aid to help make that special recipe a healthy option. Ask your dietitian for recipe suggestions so that you can occasionally include family favorites in your meal plan.

If you're going to attend a special gathering where you don't know the people well, think through what you'll eat and drink before you arrive. Consider bringing your own healthy snacks with some to share. Your dietitian can help you plan for these tempting times.

Rewards of staying on plan

Motivation to stick with your diet plan will improve as you begin to experience the benefits of your hard work:

- You'll experience fewer episodes of high and low glucose.
- You'll be better able to control your weight.
- You'll feel better and have more energy.
- You'll have greater control over your diabetes.

Questions and answers

Is it OK to drink alcohol?

Ask your doctor about appropriate alcohol intake for your specific situation. If you're having trouble controlling your blood glucose or if you have high levels of triglycerides (a type of blood fat), you may be advised to avoid alcohol. But a light to moderate amount may be fine if your diabetes is well controlled and it doesn't interfere with your medication.

In fact, a moderate intake of alcohol has been linked with a lower risk of heart disease. A moderate amount means no more than two drinks daily for men and one drink daily for women and anyone age 65 or older. One drink equals one 12-ounce can of regular beer (about 150 calories), one 5-ounce glass of wine (about 100 calories) or one $1\frac{1}{2}$-ounce shot glass of hard liquor (about 100 calories).

Always drink alcohol with a meal or with food. Never drink it instead of a meal or on an empty stomach because of the risk of low blood glucose. Remember, high-calorie beverages (especially mixed drinks that include sugary sodas and juices) can raise blood glucose and contribute to weight gain. And excessive drinking can raise your blood pressure and damage your liver.

What if I don't always follow my diet?

When you occasionally eat more food than you should or make less healthy food choices, acknowledge that it happened and move on. Don't try to skip a meal or eat less to make up for it. Just pick up with your regular meal plan and keep physically active to maintain a healthy weight.

But if you don't regularly follow a healthy-eating plan, it'll be hard to determine how much medication you need, and you may have problems with high or low blood glucose. If you have poor glucose control, you may develop serious complications (see Chapter 2). Your unhealthy habits will eventually catch up with you.

What should I eat if I'm sick?

If you can eat regular meals, stay with your usual meal plan. If you have a poor appetite but can handle some foods, try eating toast, cereal, soup, fruit juice or milk. If you can't eat any solid foods and are taking insulin or oral medications, sip on fruit juice or sugar-sweetened beverages to replace carbohydrates missed in your meals, and check with your doctor.

Will vitamins or herbal supplements help me control my diabetes?
There's not enough evidence to recommend the use of vitamins and other supplements to help control diabetes. If you're eating a nutritious diet with a variety of fruits, vegetables and whole grains every day, you're probably getting the vitamins you need. But if you're over age 50, you might consider taking a multivitamin-mineral supplement simply because aging can make it harder to absorb calcium and vitamins B-12 and D. In general, don't take supplements that exceed 100 percent of the Daily Value — check the labels.

Talk with with your doctor before taking any herbal supplement. The FDA doesn't rigorously control herbal supplements and some can be risky. In addition, some herbs have ingredients that may not mix safely with diabetes medications.

What about beverages or candies made from artificial sweeteners? Can I drink or eat them in unlimited amounts?
Most beverages and some hard candies that contain artificial sweeteners have almost no calories, and they don't count as a carbohydrate, a fat or any other exchange. Examples include:
- Acesulfame potassium (Sweet One)
- Aspartame (Equal, NutraSweet, Sweet Sprinkles)
- Saccharin (SugarTwin, Sweet-10, Sweet'n Low)
- Sucralose (Splenda)

Keep in mind that many foods labeled as *diet, dietetic* or *sugar-free* (such as sugar-free candies) contain sweeteners with calories and carbohydrates that may affect your glucose level. Check product labels for words such as *sorbitol, mannitol, xylitol, lactitol* and *maltitol*, which are sugar alcohols. Although sugar alcohols are lower in calories than sugar, don't eat unlimited quantities of sugar-free foods because other ingredients in these foods contribute calories. And in some people, as little as 20 to 50 grams of sugar alcohols can cause diarrhea, gas and bloating.

Chapter 5

Achieving a healthy weight

Being overweight is by far the greatest risk factor for type 2 diabetes. About 85 percent of people who develop this type of diabetes are overweight. By contrast, most people with type 1 diabetes are at or below their ideal weight.

Why is weight such an important factor? Fat alters how your body cells respond to the hormone insulin — it causes them to become resistant to insulin's effects, reducing the amount of blood sugar (glucose) transported into your cells. More glucose remains in your bloodstream, increasing your blood glucose level.

The good news is that you can reverse this process. As you lose weight, your cells become more responsive to insulin, allowing it to do its job. For some people with type 2 diabetes, losing weight is all that's necessary to control their diabetes and return their blood glucose to normal. And the amount of weight loss doesn't have to be extreme. A modest weight loss of 5 percent to 10 percent of your weight can lower your blood glucose level, as well as reduce your blood pressure and blood cholesterol levels.

Losing weight, as you well may know, can be a challenge. However, with a positive attitude and the right advice, it's a challenge you can meet. As you develop healthier habits, the pounds will gradually come off.

Do you need to lose weight?

Before figuring out if you're overweight by medical standards, keep in mind that many fashion models and celebrities are unrealistically thin, and you shouldn't expect to look like them. Your goal is to achieve a healthy weight — one that improves your blood glucose control and reduces your risk of other medical problems. Use your body mass index, waist circumference and personal family history to see if you could benefit from weight loss.

Body mass index

Body mass index (BMI) is a measurement based on a formula that takes into account your weight and height in determining whether you have a healthy or unhealthy percentage of body fat. To estimate your BMI, you can use the chart on the next page. Or calculate your exact BMI by using this formula:

1. Multiply your height by your height (in inches).
2. Divide your weight (in pounds) by the above results.
3. Multiply that answer by 703.

A BMI under 18.5 indicates that you're underweight, 18.5 to 24.9 is considered a healthy range, 25 to 29.9 indicates overweight, and 30 or over means you're obese.

The BMI is a helpful guide, but it's not perfect. For example, muscle weighs more than fat, and many people who are very muscular and physically fit have high BMIs without added health risks.

Waist circumference

Another way of determining if you're at a healthy weight is to measure your waist circumference. If you carry most of your weight around your waist or upper body, you have an apple shape. If you carry most of your fat around your hips and thighs, you have a pear shape. Generally, it's better to have a pear shape than an apple shape. That's because excess fat around your abdomen is linked with greater risk of weight-related diseases such as type 2 diabetes and heart disease.

To determine whether you're carrying too much weight around your abdomen, measure your waist circumference at its

What's your BMI?

To determine your body mass index (BMI), find your height in the left column. Follow that row across until you reach the column with the weight nearest yours. Look at the top of that column for your approximate BMI.

	Normal		Overweight					Obese				
BMI	19	24	25	26	27	28	29	30	35	40	45	50
Height						Weight in pounds						
4'10"	91	115	119	124	129	134	138	143	167	191	215	239
4'11"	94	119	124	128	133	138	143	148	173	198	222	247
5'0"	97	123	128	133	138	143	148	153	179	204	230	255
5'1"	100	127	132	137	143	148	153	158	185	211	238	264
5'2"	104	131	136	142	147	153	158	164	191	218	246	273
5'3"	107	135	141	146	152	158	163	169	197	225	254	282
5'4"	110	140	145	151	157	163	169	174	204	232	262	291
5'5"	114	144	150	156	162	168	174	180	210	240	270	300
5'6"	118	148	155	161	167	173	179	186	216	247	278	309
5'7"	121	153	159	166	172	178	185	191	223	255	287	319
5'8"	125	158	164	171	177	184	190	197	230	262	295	328
5'9"	128	162	169	176	182	189	196	203	236	270	304	338
5'10"	132	167	174	181	188	195	202	209	243	278	313	348
5'11"	136	172	179	186	193	200	208	215	250	286	322	358
6'0"	140	177	184	191	199	206	213	221	258	294	331	368
6'1"	144	182	189	197	204	212	219	227	265	302	340	378
6'2"	148	186	194	202	210	218	225	233	272	311	350	389
6'3"	152	192	200	208	216	224	232	240	279	319	359	399
6'4"	156	197	205	213	221	230	238	246	287	328	369	410

Source: National Institutes of Health, 1998

smallest point, usually at the level of your navel. If you're a man with a waist over 40 inches or a woman with a waist over 35 inches, you're at higher risk of health problems, especially if your BMI is 25 or higher.

Personal and family history

An evaluation of your medical history, along with that of your family, is equally important in determining if your weight is healthy.

- Do you have a health condition that would benefit from

Does your weight put you at risk of health problems?

If your BMI is 25 or over, you're at higher risk of serious health problems, such as heart disease. For Asians, a BMI of 23 or more may indicate an increased risk of health problems.

	Body mass index (BMI)	Waist measurement Men: 40 inches or less Women: 35 inches or less	Waist measurement Men: Over 40 inches Women: Over 35 inches
Overweight	25 to 29.9	Increased risk	High risk
Obese	30 to 34.9 35 to 39.9	High risk Very high risk	Very high risk Very high risk
Extremely obese	40 or over	Extremely high risk	Extremely high risk

Based on the National Institutes of Health, *The Practical Guide to Identification, Evaluation, and Treatment of Overweight and Obesity in Adults*, 2000

weight loss? For most people with type 2 diabetes, the answer to this question is yes.

- Do you have a family history of a weight-related disease or condition, such as diabetes or high blood pressure?
- Have you gained much weight since high school? Weight gain in adulthood is associated with increased health risks.
- Do you smoke cigarettes, have more than two alcoholic drinks a day or live with too much stress? In combination with these behaviors, excess weight has greater health implications.

Your results

If your BMI indicates that you aren't overweight and you're not carrying too much weight around your abdomen, there's probably no health advantage to changing your weight. Your weight is healthy.

If your BMI is 25 to 29.9 and your waist circumference exceeds healthy guidelines, you could probably benefit from losing a few pounds, especially if you answered yes to at least one personal and family health question above. Discuss your weight with your doctor during your next checkup.

If your BMI is 30 or more, losing weight can improve your over-all health and reduce your risk of serious weight-related diseases, including complications of diabetes.

Are you ready?

No one can make you lose weight. In fact, pressure from others can make matters worse. You must be internally motivated to lose weight because it's what you want.

But that doesn't mean that you have to do it all alone. Your doctor or a registered dietitian can help you develop a plan to lose weight. You can ask for support from your spouse, family and friends. You may even want to join a support group, such as Weight Watchers or Take Off Pounds Sensibly (TOPS).

To help get motivated, keep these points in mind:
- If you've just been diagnosed with a health condition, such as diabetes, now may be the right time to lose weight. Your thoughts and energies are focused on improving your health.
- To be successful, you have to believe that you can change.
- Making permanent changes in the foods that you select and eating at regular mealtimes will help you lose weight and keep it off.
- Exercise is an important part of the weight-loss process.
- If you can take pleasure in what you're doing, your chances of being successful will be much better.

Set realistic goals

Set realistic goals and start small: A weight loss of 5 percent to 10 percent of your weight in six months is a reasonable first goal for most people. Once you achieve that goal, set a new one. Another goal might be to increase your daily servings of fruits and vegetables.

Plan also for how you're going to achieve your goals — losing those 3 to 4 pounds or eating more fruits and vegetables. You might make it a goal to walk for 30 minutes five days a week or to try a new recipe each week that contains fruits or vegetables.

What's holding you back from achieving a healthy weight?

Can you identify with any of the obstacles below? If so, try the suggested strategies to increase your chances of achieving and maintaining a healthy weight.

I don't have time to make healthy meals. Healthy meals don't have to be complicated. For example, serve a fresh salad with fat-free dressing, a whole-grain roll and a piece of fruit. Stop at a deli or grocery store and buy a healthy sandwich, soup or entree that's low in calories and fat.

I don't like vegetables and fruits. Sneak them in. Add vegetables to one of your favorite soups, replace some of the meat in casseroles or pizzas with vegetables, include fresh fruit with your cereal, stir fruit into your yogurt or cottage cheese.

When eating out, I like to eat my favorite foods — not something healthy. Eat only half of your favorite foods and save the other half for the next day. (But if you dine out often, it's important to make healthy eating a regular part of your restaurant experience.) If you know that you'll be eating extra calories, increase your exercise for the day.

I can't resist certain foods that I shouldn't eat, such as chocolate and junk food. Don't keep chocolate or junk food at home. When you can't resist the urge, buy only a single serving. Have it along with your meal.

I don't like to exercise. Although exercise is important, remember that physical activity — anything that gets you moving — burns calories, too. Do activities that you enjoy.

Eating less than your calorie goal generally isn't recommended because you aren't able to eat enough food to keep you satisfied, and you're soon hungry again. Eating fewer than 1,200 calories if you're a woman or 1,400 if you're a man also can make it difficult to get enough of certain nutrients for good health.

A dietitian can help you determine a daily calorie goal to help you lose weight, taking into account a variety of factors, such as your weight, activity level, age and overall health.

All those fad diets

In general, fad diets can be risky to your health. And most people only stick with fad diets for a short while before they go off them and eventually gain their weight back.

For example, the theory behind the popular "low-carb" diets is that carbohydrates promote weight gain because rising insulin levels drive blood glucose into your cells, where it's converted into fat. In reality, carbohydrates eaten in *reasonable amounts* don't cause higher insulin levels or promote weight gain.

Although low-carbohydrate diets may result in weight loss early on, several studies confirm that this weight loss often isn't maintained. Most low-carbohydrate diets also promote foods that are high in saturated fat and trans fats and restrict disease-fighting foods such as whole grains, vegetables and fruits — this potentially increases the risk of diabetes, heart disease and some types of cancer.

So it's best to avoid fad diets and follow the advice of your doctor or dietitian.

Daily calorie goals for healthy weight loss

To lose weight, the following daily calorie goals often work well.

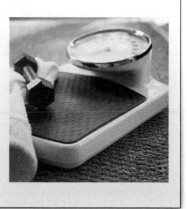

Weight	Starting calorie goal	
Pounds	*Women*	*Men*
250 or less	1,200	1,400
251 to 300	1,400	1,600
301 or more	1,600	1,800

When you achieve a goal, whether it's a weight goal or a healthy behavior goal, consider rewarding yourself with a nonfood treat.

Follow your healthy-eating plan

The same eating plan for controlling your blood glucose discussed in Chapter 4 also can help you lose weight, as long as you pay attention to the total amount of calories you consume each day. For many people, simply replacing a few servings of fats, dairy products or meat with lower calorie fruits, vegetables and whole grains is enough to reach their calorie goal.

Modifying recipes

Many recipes can be modified so that they're healthier. Experiment with some of your favorite recipes using these tips:

Reduce the amount of sugar. You can reduce the amount of sugar in most recipes by one-third to one-half of the original amount. Follow the general guideline of a quarter cup of sweetener (sugar, honey or molasses) for every cup of flour.

Use less fat. Fat in many baked products and casseroles also can be reduced by one-third to one-half. In baked goods, substitute half the shortening with applesauce or puréed fruit. Look for the words *fat-free* or *low-fat* in products such as milk, yogurt, cheese and spreads.

Make substitutions. In casseroles, cut the amount of meat in half or replace the meat with carrots, onions, lentils or beans. Replace half the flour in baked goods with whole-grain flour.

Delete an ingredient. Eliminate ingredients that are used primarily for appearance or included by habit, such as coconut, frosting and cheese, as well as condiments such as ketchup, mayonnaise and jam.

Change the method of preparation. Instead of frying, use low-fat cooking methods, such as baking, broiling, grilling, poaching or steaming.

Reduce your serving size. By eating half a serving, you consume only half the calories, sugar and fat.

Invest in a good cookbook. Visit the American Diabetes Association (ADA) Web site at *www.diabetes.org* to view cookbook titles. Also search for "Healthy Recipes Center" on *www.mayoclinic.com* — many recipes include ADA exchanges.

Small changes also add up. For example, by switching from whole milk to fat-free milk, you save 60 calories a cup. If you drink a cup of milk each day, that's 420 calories a week — that adds up to 6 pounds of weight loss in a year. If you walk 30 minutes a day at a moderate pace, you'll burn another 135 calories — and that adds up to an additional 14 pounds of weight loss in a year.

Keep a food record

Most people underestimate the number of calories they eat by at least 20 percent. Research shows that people who record the foods they eat each day often are more successful at weight loss than those who don't keep track. Each day, write down everything you eat.

You might also start a food journal. In addition to recording what you eat, you include information on when and where you eat, whether you're hungry, and your mood or feelings when you eat. You may find that certain feelings trigger particular eating behaviors. Maybe you overeat when you're depressed, angry or sad. Or maybe you eat when you're bored, even if you're not hungry.

Review your food record or journal weekly to identify potential problems or barriers to success.

Identify your unique challenges

Does your food record or journal reveal any bad habits? Maybe your problem is your simple love of particular foods, such as ice cream or salty snacks. Or perhaps you have a compulsive need to clean your plate.

If you want to beat the odds, you need to identify the factors that lead to your bad habits, and then think about how you're going to respond differently in the future. Here are some strategies that may work for you:

- Before eating anything, ask yourself if you're really hungry.
- When you have a craving for an unhealthy snack, distract yourself. Call a friend, take a walk or run an errand.
- Limit eating to the kitchen or dining room table. Don't allow yourself to eat in the living room or your bedroom, or while walking or standing around.

- When you eat, focus on eating. Don't watch TV, read or talk on the phone.
- Store food out of sight in your cupboards or refrigerator.
- Don't keep high-calorie foods around. If it's out of the house, it's out of your mouth.

Plan for difficult situations

If you're going to be in a situation that you know will be difficult for you, such as a social gathering with lots of hors d'oeuvres, develop a plan of action before you go. Eat something healthy just before you leave to decrease your hunger. Decide in advance how many hors d'oeuvres you can eat. Then eat them slowly, truly savoring the flavors. If you're still hungry, head for the vegetable tray.

Get and stay active

Eating plans that focus solely on food aren't as successful in the long term as those that combine a healthy diet and exercise. Daily exercise and increased physical activity can significantly increase your weight loss.

Exercise helps your body burn calories more efficiently, even at rest, helping you keep the pounds off. It also strengthens your body and gives you energy. And exercise can improve control of your blood glucose. For information on the benefits of exercise, see Chapter 6.

Accept and deal with setbacks

It's inevitable that you'll have setbacks, and that's OK. But don't use your setbacks as an excuse to dump your eating and activity goals. Instead, simply continue on with your plan. If you couldn't walk today because you ran out of time, walk an extra five minutes the next few days. If you ate a slice of pizza that you hadn't planned on, think about what triggered you to do so and try to learn from it.

You're not going to be perfect. Reflect on your successes, and remind yourself of the reasons you want to lose weight.

Questions and answers

I have a weakness for sweets. Can I still eat some and lose weight?
You can eat sweets once in a while without destroying your overall eating plan or interfering with your blood glucose control. It's generally best to eat them with a meal, and you need to include them in your meal plan. A dietitian can help you incorporate your favorite treats. Also, many cookbooks for people with diabetes include tasty dessert recipes.

As you acquire new eating habits, you may find that your tastes will change. Foods that you once loved may seem too sweet, and healthy substitutions may become your new idea of delicious.

Aren't some fruits and vegetables high in fat and calories?
You needn't avoid any fruits and vegetables. Although some have more calories and carbohydrates than others, you'll still benefit from the fiber and nutrients. For example, avocados are naturally higher in fat and calories than most fruits, but the fat is mostly healthy (monounsaturated fat). Just watch your intake of total calories. Refer to your diabetes exchange lists or ask your dietitian about vegetables and fruits that can be eaten in unlimited quantities and those that you need to include in your daily meal plan.

Is it OK to drink liquid meal replacement products in place of meals if I don't have time to eat?
While a healthy diet that includes whole grains, fruits and vegetables is best, a meal replacement product is a convenient alternative when eating a healthy meal isn't possible. Most meal replacement products, such as a shake or meal bar, provide fewer than 400 calories a meal and are fortified with vitamins and minerals. Ask your doctor or dietitian if meal replacement products fit into your specific meal planning.

What about prescription medications for weight loss? Can I take them if I have diabetes?
If prescription medications are indicated for weight loss, doctors generally prescribe orlistat (Xenical) or sibutramine (Meridia).

Having diabetes doesn't prevent you from taking these medications. However, the drugs aren't recommended if you have certain health conditions.

Xenical blocks the absorption of about 30 percent of dietary fat. A low-fat diet is necessary to avoid side effects such as gas, oily stools and fecal leakage. Because Xenical may reduce the absorption of fat-soluble vitamins, a daily multiple vitamin is recommended. Xenical isn't recommended for people with digestive problems.

Meridia affects chemicals in your brain, making you feel full more quickly. But this drug can increase your blood pressure and heart rate, so regular monitoring of blood pressure is important. You shouldn't take Meridia if you have heart disease, poorly controlled high blood pressure, a history of stroke, irregular heartbeat, or you're taking certain types of antidepressants. Common side effects include a dry mouth, headache, constipation and insomnia.

These medications should be used with caution and along with regular exercise and dietary changes. Average weight loss is usually modest for both products but may be enough to help improve your health. Discuss the benefits and risks of these drugs with your doctor.

I'm thinking about weight-loss surgery. Is this procedure safe for someone with diabetes?

Surgery is no easy fix for your weight problem, but sometimes it can accomplish what exercise and diet alone can't. The success of surgery depends in part on your commitment to following diet and exercise guidelines.

Surgery for weight loss is generally reserved for people who are severely overweight and have weight-related health problems, such as diabetes. Those health problems will likely improve when weight is reduced. Discuss your desire for weight-loss surgery with your doctor, who can refer you to specialists. If you're a candidate, a team of several health care professionals will evaluate you and explain the procedure, including the benefits and risks.

Chapter 6

Getting more active

Our bodies are designed to move, even if modern society makes it easy to do anything but that. You may sit at a desk all day and then come home and watch TV or put your feet up and read. It takes a special effort to incorporate exercise and other physical activity into your day. But that effort brings a bounty of health benefits — especially if you have diabetes.

The information in this chapter can help you get started on the road to a more active life. You don't have to knock yourself out to reap the benefits. Increased physical activity and a moderate amount of exercise can improve your fitness and help control your diabetes.

Physical activity vs. exercise

Physical activity refers to any body movement that burns calories, such as mowing the lawn, doing housework or climbing stairs. Exercise is a more structured form of physical activity. It involves a series of repetitive movements designed to strengthen or develop some part of your body or improve your cardiovascular fitness. Exercise includes walking, swimming, bicycling and many other activities.

Whether you're exercising or doing other types of physical activity, monitor your blood sugar (glucose) level and adjust your medications so that your glucose doesn't drop too low.

Every move counts
Regular exercise provides the greatest reward for your efforts, but you also can enjoy health benefits simply by moving around more during the day. Similar to exercise, other physical activities help lower your blood glucose, as well as your cholesterol and blood pressure.

Look for ways to build more physical activity into your day:
- Take the stairs instead of the elevator.
- Park farther from work and walk.
- Wash your car instead of taking it to the car wash.
- Walk or bike short distances instead of driving.
- Take walks with your family to explore your neighborhood.
- Walk your dog more often.
- Sweep the floors, patio and front sidewalk every day.
- Work in your garden.
- Get up to change channels on your TV instead of using the remote control.

Pedometers: Step up your health

If you need motivation to get moving, consider buying a pedometer. This small, inexpensive device detects body motion, counts steps and displays the number on a small screen. Many pedometers have additional features.

Set goals based on your fitness level and track your progress. Gradually work your way up to at least 10,000 steps a day.

Choose a pedometer that:
- Is simple to use and easy to read
- Can be read in indoor and outdoor lighting
- Is lightweight and fits snugly on your clothes
- Has a sturdy clip and a security strap so that you won't lose it

Keep in mind that a pedometer may record other movements you make (not just walking) as steps taken, making the total count at the end of the day a bit high.

Benefits of exercise

When you exercise regularly, you can:
- Improve your overall fitness, making it easier to do activities
- Reduce fatigue and increase your energy
- Improve flexibility in your muscles and joints
- Improve your muscle mass and tone
- Help prevent bone loss and osteoporosis
- Reduce your risk of high blood pressure
- Reduce stress and tension
- Reduce your risk of anxiety and depression
- Improve your concentration
- Decrease your appetite
- Improve your sense of well-being

And for people with diabetes, the benefits of regular exercise are even greater, as explained below.

Improves blood glucose control

Exercise can improve your blood glucose control by reducing your glucose level. The length and intensity of activity determines how much your glucose is lowered.

Along with a healthy-eating plan, regular exercise can reduce your need for glucose-lowering medication. In fact, some people with type 2 diabetes manage their glucose through diet and exercise alone.

Are you fit?

If you sit most of the day and get little physical activity, chances are you're not fit. Other signs that you could benefit from increased physical activity and exercise include:
- Feeling tired most of the time
- Being unable to keep up with others your age
- Avoiding physical activity because you tire easily
- Becoming short of breath or fatigued when walking a short distance or up one flight of stairs

Remember that exercise lowers your risk of disability and premature death from diabetes and many other chronic diseases.

One word of caution: Exercise can raise your blood glucose level if it's higher than 300 milligrams of glucose per deciliter of blood (mg/dL) when you begin to exercise. (See "Before exercise: Check blood glucose twice," page 99.)

Reduces risk of heart disease

Exercise is good for your heart and blood vessels. It improves the flow of blood and increases your heart's pumping power. In combination with a healthy diet, exercise also reduces low-density lipoprotein (LDL) cholesterol, the "bad" type that causes plaques to form in your blood vessels. In addition, exercise increases high-density lipoprotein (HDL) cholesterol — the "good" type that helps keep your arteries clean — and it helps lower blood pressure.

Controls your weight

Along with a healthy diet, exercise helps you lose weight and maintain a healthy weight. Regular exercise takes off pounds by burning calories and increasing your metabolism.

What type of exercise?

Aerobic exercise improves the health of your heart, lungs and circulatory system. Aerobic means "with oxygen." Aerobic activities increase your breathing and heart rate.

Aerobic activities should make up the core of your exercise program. These include activities (done at moderate intensity) such as:

- Walking
- Jogging
- Bicycling
- Aerobic dance
- Cross-country skiing
- Skating
- Tennis
- Swimming

Keep in mind that aerobic activities are endurance activities that don't require excessive speed. A higher aerobic capacity improves your endurance, making it easier for you to do household chores and climb stairs without shortness of breath.

Take a walk

Walking is one of the easiest ways to get aerobic exercise. Guidelines published by the American Association of Clinical Endocrinologists note that walking just 40 minutes four times a week is enough to lower insulin resistance, improving blood glucose control. In addition, an eight-year study of more than 70,000 women suggests that one hour a day of brisk walking may cut a woman's risk of developing type 2 diabetes almost in half.

Developing a complete fitness program

In addition to aerobic exercise, stretching and strengthening are important for good health.

Stretching exercises. Stretching before and after aerobic activity helps increase the range of motion around your joints and helps prevent joint pain and injury. But don't stretch a "cold" muscle: If you stretch before you exercise, do a short three- to five-minute warm-up first, such as low-intensity walking. If you only have time to stretch once, stretch after you exercise, when your muscles are warmed up. Stretch slowly and gently, only until you feel slight tension in your muscles.

Here are four stretches. Stretch each muscle group once. Try to do them three to five days a week and after physical activity.

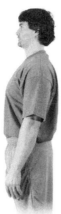 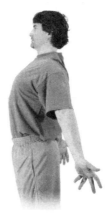

Chest stretch. Stand with arms at your sides. Then move your arms backward while rotating your palms forward as shown at right. Squeeze your shoulder blades together, breathe deeply, and lift your chest upward. Hold for 30 seconds while breathing freely, then relax. Return to start position. Repeat.

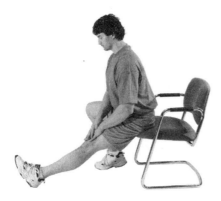

Seated hamstring stretch. Sit on a sturdy chair as shown. Maintain your normal back arch. Slowly straighten your left knee until you feel a stretch in the back of your thigh (hamstring). You may apply gentle downward pressure with your hands. Hold for 30 seconds. Relax. Repeat with the other leg.

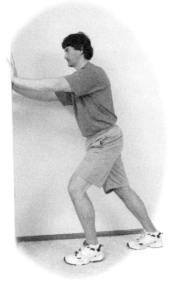

Calf stretch with straight knee. Stand at arm's length from the wall as shown. While maintaining a straight right knee (right heel on the floor), bend your left knee as if to move it toward the wall. This stretches your right calf. Hold for 30 seconds. Relax. Repeat with the other leg.

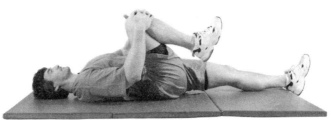

Knee-to-chest stretch.* Lie on a firm surface with your right knee bent (heel flat on the surface) and your left leg straight — or keep both knees bent if that's more comfortable. Gently pull the right knee toward your right shoulder with both hands as shown to stretch your lower back. Hold for 30 seconds. Relax. Repeat with the other leg.

*If you have osteoporosis, avoid this stretch because it can increase the risk of a compression fracture in your spine.

Strengthening exercises. Strengthening exercises build stronger muscles to improve posture, balance and coordination. They also promote healthy bones, and they increase your rate of metabolism slightly, which can help keep your weight in check.

Here are four strengthening exercises. Start with about 15 repetitions of each. Use slow and controlled motions when lifting.

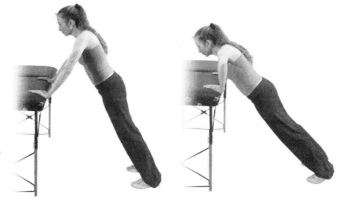

Wall or table push-ups. Lean on a wall or table as shown. Slowly bend your elbows and lean your upper body toward the wall or table, supporting your weight with your arms and keeping your heels on the floor. Straighten your arms and return to the starting position.

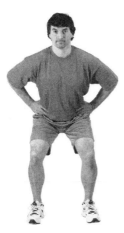

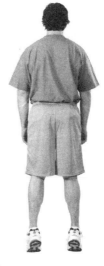

Squat. To start, stand with your feet slightly more than shoulder-width apart. Put your hands on your waist or on a table or counter. Maintaining a normal back arch, slowly bend through the hips, knees and ankles as shown. Bend your knees as far as is comfortable, but no more than 90 degrees. Keep your knees in line with your feet and not ahead of your toes. Pause, then return to the starting position.

Calf strengthening. Stand with your feet shoulder-width apart. If necessary for balance, hold on to the back of a sturdy chair. Slowly raise your heels from the floor and stand on your tiptoes. Hold. Slowly return to the starting position.

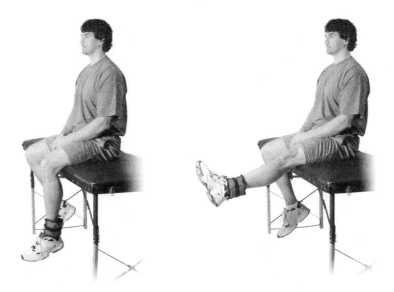

Knee extension.* Start as shown at left. Spine is in a neutral position. Maintaining alignment, slowly straighten your left knee as shown at right, pause, then return to the starting position. Do both legs. (Targets front of thighs.)

*If you have a history of knee or back pain, avoid using an ankle weight until you improve your strength. People with back problems or older adults may want to use a chair with lumbar support.

How much exercise?

Aim for at least 30 minutes of aerobic activity most days of the week. If you haven't been active for a long time, start slowly and build up your endurance. Begin by exercising 10 minutes a day. Each week, increase the length of time you exercise by five minutes, and keep adding increments.

To improve your total fitness, stretch for a few minutes after aerobic exercise to increase the flexibility in your muscles and the range of motion of your joints. Also, combine aerobic activity with strengthening exercises about two days a week.

If you don't have 30 minutes or more to exercise, break your routine into shorter intervals. You might ride a stationary bicycle for 10 to 15 minutes in the morning before going to work, walk for 10 to 15 minutes during your lunch hour and do strengthening exercises for 10 to 15 minutes in the evening.

Getting started

Before you begin a fitness program, see your doctor for a thorough medical exam. Your fitness plan should be tailored to your individual physical condition and health needs. Once you have the go-ahead from your doctor and learn if you have any limits, choose the activities for your fitness program.

Select activities you enjoy

Choose a form of exercise that fits your interests. If you like the outdoors or solitude, walking or bicycling may be good choices. If you prefer being around others, you might enjoy an aerobics class or a golf group. If you prefer watching TV or listening to music while you work out, try a stationary bicycle or treadmill.

If you have complications from your diabetes, certain types of exercise may not be good choices. For example, if you've lost feeling in your feet, swimming may be better than walking. If you have trouble seeing or have frequent episodes of low blood glucose, it may be best to exercise indoors or with a friend.

Schedule your exercise

Set aside time in your day for exercise. Write it down on your calendar or to-do list. You're more likely to make exercise a part of your daily routine if you do it at the same time each day. Of course, occasionally you'll need to reschedule or miss your exercise appointment, such as when you're sick.

Set goals and track your progress

Reaching a goal gives you encouragement. The key is to set goals that are specific and realistic. If you set a goal that's not attainable within a fairly short time, you'll be discouraged.

As your physical fitness improves, move on to a new, more challenging goal. Consider keeping a log of your progress. An exercise log helps you see what you've accomplished and helps determine your goals for the future.

Common excuses: Can you relate?
Getting started with an exercise routine can be difficult. But if you want to stay healthy, it's time to get past these excuses:

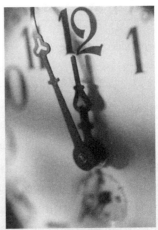

I'm too busy. If you can't manage 30 minutes at a time, break your exercise time into smaller parts — for example, three 10-minute intervals during the day. If you really want to improve your health, you can find the time.

I'm too old. You're never too old to exercise. Exercise provides benefits to all ages and may prevent or delay diseases as you get older. If you feel out of place at a health club, see if your local YMCA, YWCA or senior center offers exercise classes.

I'm too fat. Athletes may appear slim, trim and toned. But if you look around, you'll see that few people who exercise have a perfect body. Walkers, bicyclers and golfers come in all shapes and sizes. And exercise can help you achieve a healthy weight.

I'm too weak. You can start slowly and gradually increase your level of activity. The more you do, the stronger you'll begin to feel.

I'm too sick. You don't want to exercise if your blood glucose is out of control. But simply having diabetes isn't a reason to avoid exercise. Just the opposite — it's a reason to exercise. With time, exercise will help you feel better.

Vary your routine

Next to lack of motivation, boredom probably kills more exercise programs than anything else does. Keep things interesting by varying your activities and taking on more challenging ones as your physical fitness improves. You might ride a bicycle one day, walk the next, and swim another day. Include activities for all times and seasons — when you're feeling energetic, when you're not feeling as strong, when the weather is good and when it's bad.

Finding the right intensity level

Intensity refers to how hard you work when you exercise. Exercise doesn't have to be strenuous to be of benefit. You can increase your fitness with low to moderately intense exercise. Warm up before aerobic exercise and cool down afterward so that your body can gradually adjust to the changes in your activity level.

Determine if you're exercising at the right intensity level by checking your heart rate, using the perceived exertion scale or taking the talk test.

Check your heart rate

The harder you exercise, the higher your heart rate (pulse) climbs, until a maximum heart rate is reached. Most people with diabetes should exercise at a level that's 50 percent to 70 percent of their maximum heart rate. This is called your target heart rate.

If you have heart disease or other complications from diabetes, or if you take medications that affect your heart rate, ask your doctor about the appropriate target heart rate for you. If you're generally in good health, consider using these guidelines (from a study reported in the *American Journal of Cardiology*, 2001) to estimate your target heart rate range for exercising:

1. Estimate your *maximum* heart rate: Multiply your age by 0.7, then subtract that answer from 208.
2. Determine your *lower limit* heart rate: Multiply your maximum heart rate by 0.5 (50 percent of your maximum heart rate).
3. Determine your *upper limit* heart rate: Multiply your maximum heart rate by 0.7 (70 percent of your maximum heart rate).

For example, if you're 60 years old, your maximum exercise heart rate is about 166 beats a minute (60 x 0.7 = 42; 208 - 42 = 166). Your lower limit heart rate would be around 83 beats a minute (166 x 0.5). Your upper limit heart rate would be about 116 beats a minute (166 x 0.7). So your target range during exercise would be about 83 to 116 beats a minute.

Are you hitting your target range?

To estimate your heart rate while exercising, stop momentarily:

- Place two fingers on the thumb side of your wrist, press gently and feel for your pulse.
- Count your pulse for 10 seconds.
- Multiply that number by 6. This final number is your heart rate in beats per minute.

If you're just starting an exercise program, aim for the lowest part of the target range for the first few weeks and gradually work your way up. If you're on high blood pressure medications, ask your doctor if you need to lower your target heart rate range. A few high blood pressure medications might lower the maximum heart rate.

Use the perceived exertion scale

Another way to gauge the intensity of your exercise routine is to use the perceived exertion scale. Perceived exertion is the total amount of physical effort you experience during a physical activity, taking into account all sensations of exertion, physical stress and fatigue.

For an activity to produce health benefits, you need to exert a moderate to somewhat strong effort. That equates to a 3 or 4 on the perceived exertion scale. A zero rating indicates no exertion, such as when you're sitting comfortably in a chair. A 10 corresponds to maximum effort, as when jogging up a steep hill.

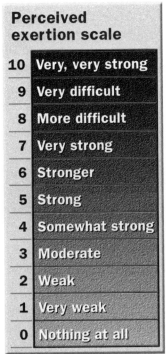

Perceived exertion scale

10	Very, very strong
9	Very difficult
8	More difficult
7	Very strong
6	Stronger
5	Strong
4	Somewhat strong
3	Moderate
2	Weak
1	Very weak
0	Nothing at all

Modified from the Borg scale, 1998

Take the talk test

While you're exercising, you should be able to carry on a short conversation without being short of breath. If you can't do this, you're probably pushing too hard and you need to slow down your pace. High-intensity exercise doesn't provide many more health benefits than moderate-intensity exercise, and it increases your risk of muscle or joint soreness and injury.

Avoiding injury

As you get more active, don't forget about safety. Follow these tips.

Wear proper clothing and shoes

Select clothes that are right for the weather and your sport. Activity increases your body temperature, so it's better to underdress than overdress. In cool weather, dress in layers so that you can remove or replace layers as you warm up or cool down. In warm weather, wear lightweight, light-colored clothes. Sweating more won't help you lose fat, just water weight, which increases your risk of overheating. Use sunscreen and wear a hat.

Make sure your shoes fit well and aren't too tight. Replace them when they begin to show signs of wear. Always put on clean, smooth-fitting socks.

Examine your feet

Check your feet before you exercise. If you see any signs of irritation, cushion the area. If you have cuts, wash them with soap and water, use an antibiotic ointment and bandage them. After exercise, check your feet again. Look for blisters, warm areas or redness.

Drink plenty of fluids

You lose fluid when you sweat, and it's important to replace this fluid. Water is the best choice. But if you're exercising for a long period, you may want the calories and electrolytes found in sports drinks. Drink fluids before, during and after exercise. The hotter the weather, the more important it is to keep your body hydrated.

Pay attention to your environment

Extreme temperatures can stress your body. On hot days, exercise indoors or during the morning or evening. In general, don't exercise outside if the temperature is higher than 80 F (27 C), especially if the humidity is high or the heat index is high. The heat index means how hot it feels like outside, based on a formula that uses both heat and humidity. Also avoid extremely cold temperatures.

Warm up and cool down

Before you begin exercising, get your body ready. Begin the exercise at a low intensity level and gradually increase the intensity level. For example, before you begin jogging or walking fast, walk for a few minutes at a slow or moderate pace to gradually increase your heart rate and oxygen flow in your lungs.

The same applies when you finish exercising — walk slowly for a while to allow your heart rate to gradually slow down. A couple of slow stretches afterward can help keep your muscles limber and prevent them from tightening up.

Heed warning signs

No matter what your workout routine, don't ignore signs and symptoms that may signal a problem, such as:

- Severe shortness of breath
- Dizziness or faintness
- Feeling sick to your stomach
- Tightness in your chest
- Chest pains
- Pain in an arm or your jaw
- Heart palpitations

Stop exercising and seek immediate medical assistance if these signs or symptoms last for more than 15 minutes. They may indicate a more serious medical problem.

Exercise and blood glucose monitoring

It's important that you track (monitor and record) your blood glucose before, during and after exercise. This helps you and your health care team to learn how your body responds to exercise.

Exercise typically reduces your blood glucose level. During exercise, glucose that's stored in your muscles and liver is used for energy. After exercise, as your body rebuilds those stores, it takes glucose from your blood, lowering your blood glucose level.

Make sure that your blood glucose isn't too low before you begin exercising and that it doesn't drop too low during and after your workout. Blood glucose monitoring can also help prevent dangerous episodes of high blood glucose and high urine ketone levels.

Before exercise: Check blood glucose twice

To avoid swings in your blood glucose, test it about 30 minutes before you start and then once again immediately before exercising. This can help you determine if your blood glucose level is stable, rising or falling before you start to exercise. Avoid problems by following these guidelines:

- **Less than 100 mg/dL.** Eat a small carbohydrate-containing snack such as fruit or crackers. Test your glucose level after 15 to 30 minutes. Wait until your glucose level is at least 100 mg/dL before starting to exercise.
- **100 to 250 mg/dL.** For most people, this is a safe pre-exercise blood glucose range.
- **250 mg/dL or higher.** Before exercising, test your urine for ketones. If the results show a moderate or high ketone level, don't exercise. Wait until your test indicates a low level of ketones. The excess ketones indicate that your body doesn't have enough insulin to control your blood glucose and this can lead to a life-threatening condition called diabetic ketoacidosis (DKA).
- **300 mg/dL or higher.** Don't exercise. You need to bring your blood glucose down before you can safely exercise because you risk an even greater increase in glucose. And high glucose levels (hyperglycemia) can lead to overproduction of urine, resulting in dehydration.

During exercise: Check blood glucose every 30 minutes

It's especially important to check your blood glucose during exercise if you're starting aerobic exercise for the first time, trying a new activity or sport, or increasing the intensity or duration of your workout. If you exercise for more than an hour, especially if you have type 1 diabetes, stop and test your blood glucose every 30 minutes.

Carry glucose sources with you to treat symptoms of low blood glucose. If your glucose is less than 100 mg/dL, or if it's not that low but you have symptoms of low blood glucose — feeling shaky, weak, anxious, sweaty or confused — eat a snack that serves as a fast-acting source of glucose.

Examples include:

- Two or three glucose tablets
- $\frac{1}{2}$ cup of fruit juice
- $\frac{1}{2}$ cup of regular (not diet) soft drink
- Five or six pieces of hard candy

Recheck your blood glucose 15 minutes after this snack. If it's still too low, have another serving and test again 15 minutes later, until your glucose reaches 100 mg/dL or higher.

When to exercise

The best time to exercise depends on your treatment. If you take insulin, avoid exercising for the three hours after injecting rapid- or short-acting insulin due to the potential risk of low blood glucose. Both insulin and exercise lower your blood glucose. Ask your doctor whether you need to adjust your insulin dose before exercising and how long you should wait to exercise after injecting insulin. Don't exercise for more than an hour unless you've discussed your insulin needs with your doctor.

If you have type 1 diabetes and you exercise for more than an hour or do strenuous activities, you may benefit from a snack before you begin or while exercising. For most people with type 2 diabetes, a snack before exercise generally isn't necessary. If you don't take medications to control your diabetes, it also may be OK to exercise after you eat, when your blood glucose level is generally highest.

After exercise: Check blood glucose at least twice

The more strenuous the workout, the longer your blood glucose is affected. Check your blood glucose a couple of times after exercising to make sure you aren't developing hypoglycemia, which can occur even hours after you've stopped.

Be patient

You may think that testing your blood glucose before, during and after you exercise requires a lot of effort. But once you know how your body responds to exercise, you may not need to check your blood glucose as often — follow your doctor's advice.

Questions and answers

What if I have a lapse in my routine?

It happens to everyone. You're swamped with work, on vacation or sick, and your exercise plan flies out the window. Everyone who follows a long-term exercise program has off days. Don't be too critical — remind yourself it's only a temporary setback. As soon as possible, try to resume your regular exercise schedule.

What if I don't feel like exercising?

There will be days when that will happen. Maybe you had a hard day at work, or you're dead tired or just not in the mood. On these days, try the five-minute compromise. Tell yourself that you'll exercise for just five minutes. If you don't feel like continuing after five minutes, you can stop and not feel guilty about it. Nine times out of 10, once you've started, you'll want to continue.

What if I drink alcohol and exercise?

When you mix alcohol and exercise, you increase your risk of low blood glucose. Exercise and alcohol both tend to lower blood glucose. It's best not to drink alcohol during or after exercise. If you do, have some food with your drink. (See "Is it OK to drink alcohol?" page 71.)

If I'm active on my job, do I need an exercise program?

If your job is truly active — you're constantly moving eight to 10 hours a day — such physical activity can certainly benefit your health by burning calories. However, work-related activity generally doesn't offer the same level of health benefits that exercise does. For example, structured exercises can focus on strengthening specific parts of your body, improve your cardiovascular fitness and help reduce stress.

Part 3

Medical treatments

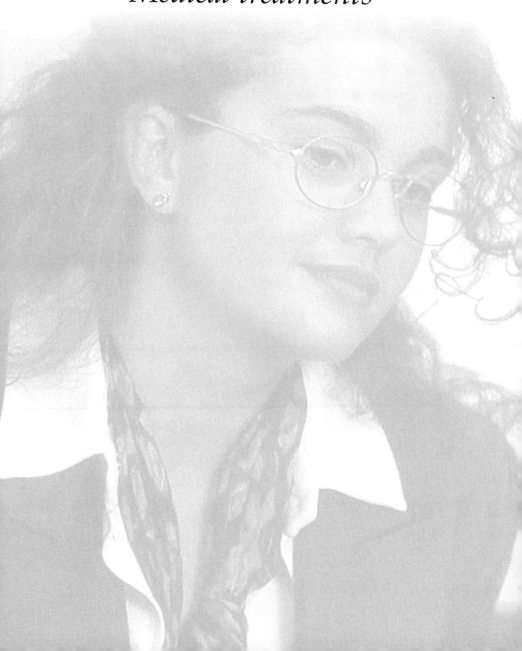

Chapter 7

Insulin therapy

I f you have type 1 diabetes, you need insulin injections to replace the insulin your pancreas no longer produces. If you have type 2 diabetes and don't benefit from other medications, you also may need to take insulin.

Treatment with insulin, called insulin therapy, has two main goals:

1. To maintain blood sugar (glucose) at near-normal levels or within the target range that your doctor recommends
2. To prevent long-term complications of diabetes

The most widely used form of insulin is synthetic human insulin, which is chemically identical to human insulin but manufactured in a laboratory. Some insulins, known as insulin analogs, are modified by the manufacturer to better mimic normal insulin secretion by the pancreas.

Your doctor can help you decide which insulin treatment works best for you. That will depend on:

- Trends and patterns of your blood glucose levels
- Your lifestyle
- What you eat
- How much you exercise
- Whether or not you have other health conditions

Pramlintide (Symlin)

In addition to insulin, another treatment for type 1 diabetes is pramlintide (Symlin), recently approved by the Food and Drug Administration. Pramlintide is only for adults with type 1 or type 2 diabetes who use insulin and need better control of their blood glucose. Taken as an injection before you eat, pramlintide can help lower blood glucose during the three hours after meals. For more on this drug, see Chapter 8, page 136.

Types of insulin

Many types of insulin are available. They differ in the time it takes to begin working (onset), at what point the insulin has the most effect on glucose (peak) and how long the overall effect lasts (duration). Insulin is administered by an injection or through continuous infusion from an insulin pump. You and your health care team will determine the type and amount of insulin that best meets your needs. See the "Insulin options" chart on page 108.

What is premixed insulin?

Premixed insulin combines rapid- or short-acting insulin with intermediate-acting insulin. This is convenient if you need two types of insulin but have trouble drawing up insulin out of two bottles, or you have poor eyesight or arthritis or other problems with your hands. But available products may not match your specific needs.

There are several premixed insulins, and some have long generic names. The numbers after each brand name show that the bottle contains two types of insulin in different percentages (such as 50 percent intermediate-acting insulin and 50 percent short-acting insulin): Humulin 50/50, Humulin 70/30, Novolin 70/30, NovoLog Mix 70/30, Humalog Mix 75/25 and ReliOn/Novolin 70/30.

Because you're getting two different types of insulin, the onset, peak and duration of each type will differ but overlap. Follow the directions of your doctor or diabetes educator, but typically if the premixed product has short-acting insulin, you'll inject it 30 minutes before a meal; if the premixed product has rapid-acting insulin, you'll inject it no more than 15 minutes before your meal.

Insulin regimens

Options for insulin regimens include:

Single dose. You inject a dose of intermediate-acting or long-acting insulin once each day.

Mixed dose. You inject rapid- or short-acting insulin and intermediate-acting insulin — mixed in one syringe.

Premixed dose. You inject a dose of premixed insulin once or twice a day.

Split dose. You give yourself two injections of intermediate-acting insulin each day. These injections are usually given before breakfast and before the evening meal, or before breakfast and at bedtime.

Split mixed dose. You give yourself two injections that contain a combination of a rapid- or short-acting insulin and an intermediate-acting insulin — mixed in one syringe — each day. These are generally given before breakfast and before the evening meal.

Split premixed dose. You give yourself two injections of premixed insulin daily. These are usually given before breakfast and before the evening meal.

Intensive insulin therapy. This regimen involves multiple daily injections of insulin or using a small portable pump that continuously administers insulin.

Intensive insulin therapy

People taking insulin have less risk of complications from their diabetes if they can keep their blood glucose within a normal or near-normal range (tight glucose control). For people with type 1 diabetes, the preferred form of therapy to achieve this is intensive insulin therapy. People with type 2 diabetes can benefit from intensive insulin therapy if oral medications, other insulin regimens and lifestyle changes don't keep blood glucose levels in the target range.

Intensive insulin therapy involves monitoring your blood glucose frequently, using a combination of insulins and adjusting your insulin doses based on your blood glucose levels, your diet and changes in your routine. When practiced effectively, intensive insulin therapy can greatly lower your risk of complications.

Insulin options

You and your health care team will determine the type and amount of insulin that best meets your needs. Below are examples, but talk with your doctor and check the package insert of the product for complete information. Keep in mind that:

Type of insulin	Insulin name (brand name)	Onset of action
Rapid-acting Absorbed more quickly than short-acting insulin and effects wear off sooner	insulin aspart (NovoLog) insulin glulisine (Apidra) insulin lispro (Humalog)	10 to 30 minutes (range varies by product)
Short-acting Works quickly, but effects don't last as long as intermediate-acting insulin	insulin regular (Humulin R, Novolin R, ReliOn/Novolin R)	30 to 60 minutes
Intermediate-acting Starts working later than short-acting insulin and effects last longer	NPH[†] (Humulin N, Novolin N, ReliOn/Novolin N)	1 to 2 hours
Long-acting Takes several hours to work, but provides insulin at a steady level for up to 24 hours	insulin glargine (Lantus)	1 to 5 hours
	insulin detemir (Levemir), available in 2006	Data not available

†NPH stands for neutral protamine Hagedorn.

- *Onset of action* means how soon the insulin starts to lower blood glucose.
- *Peak action* means when the insulin works the strongest.
- *Duration* means how long the overall effect lasts.

Peak action	Duration	How it's typically used*
30 minutes to 3 hours (range varies by product)	3 to 5 hours (range varies by product)	Inject immediately before a meal — can cause blood glucose to drop too low (hypoglycemia) if injected too early before a meal. Often used in addition to intermediate- or long-acting insulin.
2 to 5 hours (range varies by product)	Up to 8 hours (range varies by product)	Inject 30 minutes before a meal. May be used in addition to intermediate- or long-acting insulin.
4 to 12 hours (range varies by product)	16 to 24 hours (range varies by product)	Generally covers insulin needs for about half a day. Should last overnight when used just before bedtime. May be used in addition to rapid- or short-acting insulin.
No clear peak	Up to 24 hours	Effects last for about a day. *Should not be mixed* with other types of insulin in one syringe but may be used in addition to rapid- or short-acting insulin. *Don't* use in insulin pumps.
No clear peak	Up to 24 hours	

*Follow the advice of your doctor. Onset, peak and duration times are estimates — times vary among individuals and are affected by the site of injection and other issues, such as when you last ate or exercised.

Sources: Product manufacturers and *Pharmacist's Letter/Prescriber's Letter*, August 2005

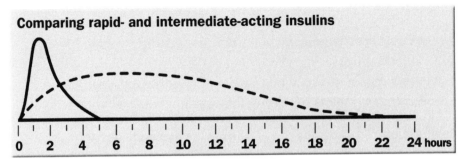

Comparing rapid- and intermediate-acting insulins

This shows an example of the difference between rapid-acting (solid line) and intermediate-acting (broken line) insulins in time of onset, peak and duration.

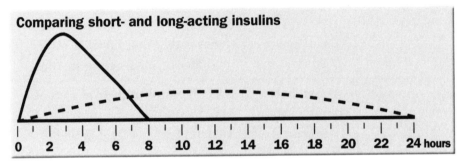

Comparing short- and long-acting insulins

This shows an example of the difference between short-acting (solid line) and long-acting (broken line) insulins in time of onset, peak and duration.

If your doctor recommends intensive insulin therapy, there are two options:

Multiple daily injections. You take three or more injections of insulin each day to achieve tight control of your blood glucose. You may take an injection of rapid- or short-acting insulin before meals as well as an injection of intermediate- or long-acting insulin once daily.

Insulin pump. An insulin pump continuously releases rapid- or short-acting insulin into your body through a plastic tube placed underneath the skin on your abdomen. (See "How insulin pumps work" on page 119 for more details.)

Drawbacks of intensive insulin therapy

Intensive insulin therapy has two possible drawbacks: low blood glucose (hypoglycemia) and weight gain. When your blood glucose is already close to normal, hypoglycemia can occur even with minor changes in your routine, such as an unexpected increase in activity. You can counter this risk by being aware of changes in your routine that increase your risk of hypoglycemia. It's also important to recognize the signs and symptoms of low blood glucose and respond quickly when you begin to experience them. (See "Low blood glucose," page 22.)

Weight gain can occur because the more insulin you use to control your blood glucose, the more glucose that gets into your cells

Tight glucose control: Preventing complications

Several studies confirm that tight blood glucose control — keeping your blood glucose within a normal or near-normal range — can dramatically reduce your risk of developing complications.

Diabetes Control and Complications Trial

In the 10-year Diabetes Control and Complications Trial (DCCT), more than 1,400 volunteers with type 1 diabetes were randomly assigned to one of two groups:

1. The conventional group received routine insulin therapy as advised by their doctors to control their blood glucose.
2. The intensive therapy group received intensive insulin therapy using injections or an insulin pump. Their goal was to keep their blood glucose as close to normal as possible.

Results showed that tight blood glucose control using intensive insulin therapy reduced the risk of many complications — such as eye damage or kidney disease — by at least 50 percent compared with those receiving conventional treatment.

United Kingdom Prospective Diabetes Study

The United Kingdom Prospective Diabetes Study (UKPDS) recruited more than 5,100 people with newly diagnosed type 2 diabetes. Participants were followed for an average of 10 years.

The results showed that, overall, people who tried to keep their blood glucose at a normal level had one-fourth fewer complications involving their eyes, kidneys and nerves. Improved blood glucose and blood pressure control also led to a reduced risk of heart disease.

and the less glucose that's wasted in your urine. Glucose that your cells don't use accumulates as fat. Following a healthy-eating plan can help limit weight gain.

Work with your health care team

Talk with your doctor to find out if intensive insulin therapy is for you. You'll probably measure your blood glucose level more often,

---

Alternatives to the syringe and needle

The insulin pen and insulin jet injector are options to the syringe and needle for insulin delivery. An insulin pump (see page 119) is another alternative. All options have pros and cons. Discuss them with your doctor to determine which method is best for you. And find out what your insurance covers before you buy.

Insulin pen. This device looks like a pen with a cartridge. Refillable pens have pre-filled disposable cartridges that contain insulin. Other pens are completely disposable. You place a fine-point needle, much like the one on a syringe, on the tip of the pen. You turn a dial to select the desired insulin dose, insert the needle under your skin and click down on a button at the end of the pen to deliver the insulin.

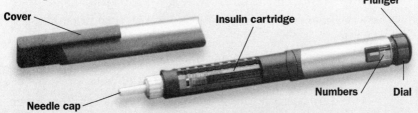

Cover · Insulin cartridge · Plunger · Numbers · Dial · Needle cap

Refillable injection pen

If you have arthritis, a disposable insulin pen is convenient because you won't have to load and unload insulin cartridges. A disposable insulin pen with large numbers on the dial may work best if you have vision problems.

Insulin jet injector. This device uses high-pressure air to send a fine spray of insulin under your skin. There may be some discomfort and possible bruising. This device may not be as accurate as other methods because some of the insulin can be lost during injection. Jet injectors are more expensive than pen injectors.

and if you take insulin, your health care team may change your schedule. But remember that healthy eating and exercising also are vital for glucose control. Think of tight glucose control and a healthy lifestyle as key factors that can add many healthy years to your life.

How to inject insulin

When first diagnosed with diabetes, you may feel frightened or nervous about injecting yourself with insulin. That's natural. Learning about the process and doing it a few times will help you feel more comfortable. The most common way to receive insulin is by syringe. This method delivers insulin underneath the skin, where it's absorbed into the bloodstream.

Selecting a site

Insulin may be injected into any area of your body where a layer of fatty tissue is present and where large blood vessels, nerves, muscles and bones aren't close to the surface.

Insulin is best injected into the abdomen because of quick and consistent absorption. Avoid the two-inch radius around the navel, which doesn't absorb as well. Rotate the site of each injection as shown in the illustration at right. Your doctor or diabetes educator may recommend alternative areas for injection, such as your upper arms, thighs or buttocks.

After you determine the site for your insulin injection, clean it with an alcohol wipe or soap and water, and allow it to dry before giving yourself an injection.

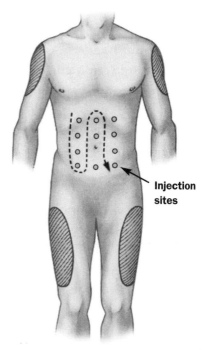

Injection sites

Generally the abdomen is the best injection site. Rotate the site of each injection. The upper arms and thighs (shaded areas) as well as the buttocks also are potential injection sites.

Drawing insulin into a syringe

With time and practice the process of drawing insulin into a syringe becomes routine and is no longer so daunting. Here's how to do it:

1. Gather your supplies: bottle of insulin, syringe and needle, alcohol wipe and a covered, puncture-resistant container for needle discard.

2. Check the label on the insulin bottle for the type, concentration and expiration date. Use the same type of insulin every time, unless your doctor tells you otherwise. Changing insulin types may affect blood glucose control.

3. Check the insulin bottle for any changes in the insulin. Make sure no clumping, frosting, precipitation or change in clarity or color has occurred, which may mean that the insulin has lost potency.

4. Wash your hands with soap and water.

5. Clear insulin doesn't need to be mixed. However, cloudy insulin should be mixed by gently rolling the bottle between your hands. (Don't shake the bottle — that may decrease the insulin's potency.) Then, check to make sure there are no particles at the bottom of the bottle.

6. Wipe off the top of the insulin bottle with an alcohol wipe.

7. Remove the needle cap from the sterile syringe.

8. Pull the plunger to draw in an amount of air equal to the amount of insulin that you need.

9. Insert the needle through the rubber stopper of the insulin bottle and push the plunger so air goes into the bottle. This equalizes air pressure in the bottle, making it easier to withdraw the insulin.

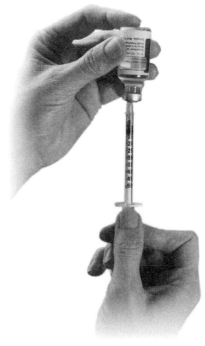

10. While keeping the needle in the bottle, turn the bottle upside down.
11. Pull the plunger on the syringe and withdraw insulin, not air, slightly past the number of units needed. Air isn't dangerous but it reduces the amount of insulin in the syringe.
12. If there are air bubbles, remove them. Either push the insulin back into the bottle (without taking the needle out of the bottle) and draw it again, or snap the syringe sharply with your finger and then push the plunger to expel the air into the bottle.
13. Recheck the syringe for air. If air is present, repeat the previous step.
14. Double-check the amount of insulin in the syringe.
15. Pull the needle out of the bottle.

It may seem like a lot of steps to prepare for the injection, but once you become comfortable with injecting yourself, it takes very little time.

Injecting the insulin

Once you have the right amount of insulin in the syringe and you've removed the needle from the bottle, it's time to inject the insulin:

- Hold the syringe like a pencil. Quickly insert the entire length of the needle into a fold of your skin at a 90-degree angle as shown in the illustration. (If you're thin, you may need to use a short needle or inject at a 45-degree angle to avoid injecting into your muscle, especially in the thigh area.)
- Release the pinched skin. Inject the insulin by gently pushing the plunger all the way down at a steady, moderate rate, and pause for five seconds before withdrawing the needle from your skin. (If the plunger jams as you're injecting the insulin, remove the needle and note the number of units remaining in the syringe. Contact your doctor or diabetes educator for advice.)

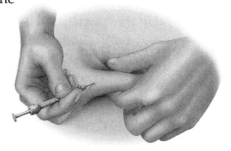

- Don't re-cap the needle. Discard it in a covered, puncture-resistant container.

Mixing two different types of insulin

If you need to inject two types of insulin at the same time (rapid- or short-acting with intermediate-acting insulin), follow the procedure below. Note: *Never* mix long-acting insulin — insulin glargine (Lantus) or insulin detemir (Levemir) — with other types of insulin. *Always draw the rapid- or short-acting insulin into the syringe first.*

Write down the amount of each type of insulin. Add the two numbers together to determine the total number of units. Follow steps No. 1 through No. 7 on page 114, "Drawing insulin into a syringe." From there, you:

1. Pull the plunger to draw in an amount of air equal to the amount of intermediate-acting insulin that you need.
2. Insert the needle through the rubber stopper of the intermediate-acting insulin bottle and push the plunger so that air goes into the bottle to equalize the air pressure in the bottle.
3. Pull the needle out of the bottle *without withdrawing any insulin.*
4. Pull the plunger to draw in an amount of air equal to the amount of short- or rapid-acting insulin you need.
5. Insert the needle through the rubber stopper on the short- or rapid-acting insulin bottle and push the plunger so that air goes into the bottle.
6. While keeping the needle in the bottle, turn the bottle upside down.
7. Pull the plunger on the syringe and withdraw insulin, not air, slightly past the number of units needed.

Avoid injection site problems

Occasionally, especially when you first start using insulin, you may notice redness and slight swelling at the injection site. It could be the result of impurities in the insulin, or it could stem from a small amount of alcohol getting into fat tissues. To avoid this, let the injection site dry after cleaning it with alcohol. If the skin irritation lasts more than two to three weeks or causes you discomfort, talk with your doctor.

8. If there are air bubbles, remove them. Either push the insulin back into the bottle (without taking the needle out of the bottle) and draw it again, or snap the syringe sharply with your finger and then push the plunger to expel the air into the bottle.
9. Recheck the syringe for air. If air is present, repeat the previous step.
10. Double-check the amount of insulin in the syringe.
11. Pull the needle out of the bottle.
12. Insert the needle through the rubber stopper of the intermediate-acting insulin bottle.
13. While keeping the needle in the bottle, turn the bottle upside down.
14. Carefully withdraw the required number of insulin units. If you draw more than the correct amount, don't push the insulin back into the bottle. Throw away the syringe and begin again.
15. Double-check the amount of insulin in the syringe. It should equal the total number of units that you wrote down.
16. Pull the needle out of the bottle. To finish the procedure, see "Injecting the insulin," page 115.

If you have trouble mastering the mixing technique, ask someone on your health care team to demonstrate the procedure or to observe and coach you as you go through the steps. Or ask your doctor whether premixed insulin is an option for you. (See "What is premixed insulin?" page 106.)

To minimize painful injections, remember these tips:
• Make sure the insulin is at room temperature.
• Be sure no air bubbles are in the syringe.
• Relax your muscles in the area of the injection.
• Penetrate your skin quickly with the needle.
• Don't change the direction of the needle during the injection.
Some people develop indentations, hard lumps or thickened skin in areas where they inject insulin — avoid injecting in these

Avoiding problems with insulin

The following steps can reduce your risk of problems from insulin use:

Buy all of your insulin from the same pharmacy. This will help ensure that you receive the type and concentration of insulin that's prescribed and alert you to changes in your prescription. Check the expiration date on the package and always keep a spare bottle on hand.

Store your insulin in the refrigerator until it's opened. After a bottle has been opened, it may be kept at room temperature for one month. Insulin at room temperature causes less discomfort when injected. Throw away your insulin after the expiration date or after being kept at room temperature for a month.

Avoid temperature extremes. Never freeze insulin or expose it to extremely hot temperatures or direct sunlight.

Look for changes in appearance. Throw away insulin that is discolored or contains solid particles.

Wear diabetes identification. Wear an identification necklace or bracelet that identifies you as an insulin user. In addition, carry an identification card that includes the name and phone number of your doctor and all the medications you're taking, including the kind of insulin. In case your blood glucose drops too low, this will help people know how to respond.

Speak up. To avoid possible drug interactions or drug side effects, inform your dentist, pharmacist and those doctors who may not be familiar with your medical history that you take insulin.

Check all medications. Before taking any medication other than your insulin, including over-the-counter products, read the warning label. If the label says you shouldn't take the drug if you have diabetes, consult your doctor before taking it.

Get help for allergic reactions. In rare instances, insulin injections may cause breathing or swallowing problems. If this happens, you may be having a potentially life-threatening allergic reaction called anaphylaxis (an-uh-fuh-LAK-sis). This is a medical emergency — go to an emergency room immediately.

areas because insulin won't be absorbed well. Rotating the site of your injections may prevent or reduce this problem.

How insulin pumps work

An insulin pump is a computerized device that's about the size of a pager or small cell phone. It can be worn on your belt or in your pocket. The pump provides a continuous supply of insulin, eliminating the need for daily shots. It has a container that you fill with insulin. A small, flexible tube connects the container of insulin to a catheter that's inserted under the skin of your abdomen. You use a needle to insert the catheter and then withdraw the needle.

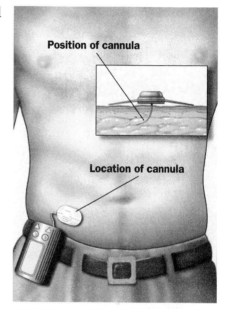

Insulin pumps deliver a continuous drip of insulin through a tube (cannula) inserted under the skin of your abdomen.

Based on information that you program into the device, the pump delivers a continuous (basal) infusion of short- or rapid-acting insulin and extra insulin (a bolus) before meals to cover an expected rise in blood glucose from the meals.

Every second or third day you need to change the infusion site. To do this, you pull out the catheter and insert a new one at a different site. Your doctor or diabetes educator will likely recommend that you rotate the injection site among the four quadrants of your abdomen. The reservoir that holds the insulin also needs to be refilled every few days.

If you decide to use an insulin pump, you'll typically go through thorough training in all aspects of pump use and intensive diabetes management. During this training you'll learn how to determine your insulin requirements, how to program your pump to safely administer the insulin and how to insert the catheter and care for the injection site.

Convenience and control

Several studies confirm the effectiveness of pump therapy, known as continuous subcutaneous insulin infusion (CSII). The main advantage of insulin pumps is improved blood glucose control. People who use insulin pumps are often able to achieve normal or near-normal blood glucose levels.

Today's pumps are smaller than a deck of cards. Many people feel a pump allows a more flexible lifestyle. Other advantages include:

- Built-in safety alarms to let you know if the line's plugged, you're out of insulin or the battery is low
- Memory display of previous insulin delivery
- The ability to program different rates of insulin delivery to help prevent low blood glucose (hypoglycemia) and high blood glucose (hyperglycemia)
- The ability to control meal-related insulin delivery
- The ability to suspend or decrease insulin delivery during exercise and physical activity
- Quick release technology to easily disconnect the infusion tubing for situations such as showering, swimming or engaging in sexual activity
- Better blood glucose control in hard-to-control situations: travel, variable work shifts, erratic schedules

Who's a candidate?

Insulin pumps can be beneficial, but they aren't for everybody. If you're doing a good job of controlling your diabetes without a pump, the investment may not bring significant improvements in blood glucose control or your lifestyle.

To benefit from a pump you need to use it properly, monitor your blood glucose regularly and be willing to work closely with your doctor and diabetes educator. Some people find this regimen too demanding. The pumps also are expensive, costing up to several thousand dollars. Many times, though, this cost is covered, at least in part, by insurance. Other drawbacks include risk of infection at the pump site, high blood glucose if the pump fails to deliver insulin, and difficulty incorporating the pump into physical activities, such as contact sports.

Some women with diabetes who are pregnant or are trying to become pregnant prefer an insulin pump. High blood glucose in early pregnancy can cause birth defects and illness in infants. Tight control of blood glucose reduces that risk. An insulin pump also may benefit people with:

Poor blood glucose control despite multiple injection therapy. Insulin pump therapy can match the insulin needs of some people better than insulin injections can. Frequent blood glucose monitoring helps determine your insulin needs.

Episodes of severe low blood glucose. A pump can reduce the incidence of severe hypoglycemia.

Extreme insulin sensitivity. A pump can deliver very small amounts of insulin at a time, which is hard to do with injections.

Problems of dawn phenomenon. Some people experience increased glucose production in the early morning hours, called the dawn phenomenon, and need more insulin at that time. You can program your pump to increase insulin delivery during that time.

Variable work or activity schedules. A pump allows you the freedom to program your insulin doses to meet your changing needs.

Use the pump correctly

You need to know how your pump works and not be afraid of mechanical devices. It's essential that you have a clear understanding of the relationship between insulin, food and activity so that you can program your pump to help you in changing situations. Even when using a pump, you still need to check your blood glucose four or more times a day. It's also important to meet regularly with your doctor or diabetes educator to make sure you're using the device correctly and all is going well.

Implantable insulin pumps

An implantable insulin pump system is being clinically evaluated but not yet available for public use in the United States. Implanting an insulin pump in your lower abdomen may be more convenient and less noticeable. The pump delivers small amounts of insulin throughout the day, which may help people who have a difficult time maintaining good glucose control.

Questions and answers

What should I do if I forget to give myself an insulin injection?
If you miss just one dose, it's generally not a problem. Wait until the next scheduled time for an injection and give yourself the regular amount. Don't double it to make up for the missed injection.

If I'm sick, especially if I'm vomiting, do I still take my usual doses of insulin?
Continue to take insulin, especially if you have type 1 diabetes, to prevent significant blood glucose elevations or accumulation of blood acids (ketoacidosis). Monitor your blood glucose frequently and adjust your insulin doses as necessary. Keep well hydrated by drinking fluids that contain calories. If your blood glucose is consistently above 300 mg/dL or you're unable to keep fluids down because of vomiting, call your doctor.

If I'm scheduled for surgery, do I take my insulin as usual?
Before surgery you'll be fasting. If you're injecting insulin, usually you'll be told to omit the rapid-acting and short-acting doses. The general rule of thumb is to take half of your usual intermediate-acting dose or your usual long-acting dose, but verify this with your doctor. If you're using a pump, typically you'll be told to keep the basal insulin dose going. Your doctor may make other adjustments to your insulin delivery before and during surgery until you can safely resume this responsibility.

Are researchers working on other ways to deliver insulin?
Researchers continue to explore new methods of insulin delivery, such as patches, pills, an oral spray, and an artificial pancreas that's placed into the abdomen and releases insulin as needed.

An inhaled form of insulin may be nearing FDA approval. Using an inhalation device, the powdered insulin is inhaled through your mouth into your lungs before eating. However, early studies show a small decline in lung function in some people, which may worsen symptoms in those with asthma or other lung disorders.

Chapter 8

Medications
for type 2 diabetes

I f you have type 2 diabetes, there are several approaches to help manage your blood sugar (glucose). Although many people can control type 2 diabetes by proper eating, exercise and maintaining a healthy weight, lifestyle changes alone aren't enough for some people. You may need medications to help control your blood glucose — but remember that a healthy diet and regular exercise still play a key role.

Options for the medical treatment of type 2 diabetes include:
- Medications taken by mouth (oral drugs)
- Insulin
- New injectable drugs

Your doctor may recommend more than one drug, or you may need to take drugs along with insulin. Most people begin with an oral drug.

Oral drugs

Several classes of oral drugs are available. Each class has a different chemical structure and its own method for lowering blood glucose. Some oral medications stimulate your pancreas to release more insulin, others make your body's cells more sensitive to the effects of insulin, and still others slow your body's absorption of carbohydrates.

Oral drugs for type 2 diabetes

Each class of drugs that manage blood glucose works differently, and some drugs aren't for use in young children. Here are the main advantages and disadvantages — see pages 126 to 131 for more details. Your doctor may recommend one or more

Drug class Drug name (brand name)	How they work
Sulfonylureas* glimepiride** (Amaryl) glipizide** (Glucotrol, Glucotrol XL) glyburide** (DiaBeta, Glynase, Micronase)	Stimulate your pancreas to release more insulin
Biguanides metformin** (Fortamet, Glucophage, Glucophage XR, Riomet)	Reduce the amount of glucose your liver releases into your bloodstream between meals
Alpha-glucosidase inhibitors acarbose (Precose) miglitol (Glyset)	Slow absorption of glucose into your bloodstream after eating carbohydrates
Thiazolidinediones, **also called TZDs** pioglitazone (Actos) rosiglitazone (Avandia)	Help reduce blood glucose by making body tissues more sensitive to insulin (may take a few weeks to notice effect on blood glucose)
Meglitinides nateglinide (Starlix) repaglinide (Prandin)	Stimulate your pancreas to release more insulin when glucose levels rise after a meal

*Acetohexamide, chlorpropamide (Diabinese), tolazamide (Tolinase) and tolbutamide are some of the first sulfonylureas put on the market, but now they're rarely used because they typically have more side effects than the newer drugs.

**These drugs are also available in generic form, which usually costs less.

medications. Talk with your doctor or pharmacist before taking any over-the-counter or prescription drug. It's best to have all of your prescriptions filled at the same pharmacy so that your pharmacist can alert you to any potential drug interactions.

Main advantages	Main disadvantages
Work well with other oral diabetes drugs for added effectiveness to lower blood glucose	Can cause abnormally low blood glucose (hypoglycemia)
Does not cause hypoglycemia; may promote weight loss; may reduce blood fats (cholesterol and triglycerides)	Can cause nausea, upset stomach and diarrhea (typically resolves over time); rare, serious side effect is lactic acidosis (lactic acid builds up in your body)
Limits rapid rise of blood glucose that can occur after meals (taken with meals); may promote weight loss	Can cause abdominal bloating and discomfort, gas and diarrhea, so start in smaller doses; high doses can harm your liver; less effective on lowering blood glucose than other oral drugs
Convenient: taken once or twice a day with or without food; not linked with stomach upset when used alone	Can cause side effects such as swelling (edema) and weight gain that may lead to or worsen heart failure; require close monitoring for liver problems; may lessen effects of birth control pills
Work quickly when taken with meals to reduce high glucose levels; less likely than sulfonylureas to cause hypoglycemia	Effects wear off quickly and drugs must be taken with each meal; can cause upset stomach and hypoglycemia

Which drug is best?

Talk with your doctor and diabetes educator about the pros and cons of each drug — they'll recommend an option based on your specific needs. The box on pages 124 and 125 lists several classes of drugs, with examples of the main advantages and disadvantages. Decisions are based on several factors, such as:

- Whether you're overweight (some diabetes drugs cause weight gain)
- Your blood glucose levels and when they tend to rise (after meals, for example)
- Whether you have additional health problems
- Strength (potency) of the drug
- Possible side effects
- Cost, especially when several medications are needed (See "How can I keep my medication costs down?" page 138.)

Sulfonylureas

Sulfonylureas (sul-fuh-nil-yoo-REE-uhs) have been used for decades to control blood glucose. The drugs work by stimulating beta cells in your pancreas to produce more insulin. So, to benefit from the medication, your pancreas must be able to produce some insulin on its own.

Glimepiride (Amaryl and generic), glipizide (Glucotrol and generic) and glyburide (DiaBeta, Glynase, Micronase and generic) are the most commonly used sulfonylureas. Glipizide is available in two forms: a short-acting version and a sustained-release (XL) version. Other sulfonylureas, listed in the footnote on page 124, tend to have more side effects.

Possible side effects

Low blood glucose (hypoglycemia) is a common side effect of sulfonylureas. You're at a much greater risk of developing hypoglycemia if you have impaired liver or kidney (renal) function. If you have one of these conditions, your doctor may decide not to prescribe a sulfonylurea.

Precautions

Doing anything that reduces your blood glucose after you've taken a sulfonylurea, such as skipping a meal or exercising more than usual, can lead to low blood glucose. Taking alcohol or certain drugs with sulfonylureas, including decongestants, also can cause low blood glucose by boosting the effects of the medication. Medications such as steroids and niacin can decrease the effectiveness of sulfonylureas.

Biguanides

Biguanides (bi-GWAH-nides) improve your body's response to insulin, decreasing insulin resistance. Between meals your liver releases stored glucose into your bloodstream. Often too much glucose is released in people with type 2 diabetes. Biguanides reduce the amount of glucose your liver releases during fasting. As a result, you need less insulin to transport glucose from your blood to your individual cells.

Metformin (Glucophage and generic) is the only drug in this class available in the United States. Metformin is also available in extended release pills (Fortamet, Glucophage XR and generic) and in liquid form (Riomet). An important benefit of the drug is that it's associated with less weight gain than other diabetes medications and it may promote weight loss. For this reason, it's often prescribed to overweight or obese people with type 2 diabetes. In addition, the drug may reduce blood fats (cholesterol and triglycerides), which tend to be higher than normal in people with type 2 diabetes.

Possible side effects

Metformin is generally well tolerated, but it can produce side effects in some people. Let your doctor know if you experience any of the following:

- Loss of appetite
- Nausea or vomiting
- Gas or diarrhea
- Abdominal bloating, discomfort or pain
- Changes in taste, such as an unpleasant metallic taste in your mouth

These effects usually occur during the first few weeks of taking the medication and decrease with time. They're less likely to occur if you take the medication with food and if you start out at a low dose and gradually increase the amount you take.

A rare but serious side effect of metformin is lactic acidosis, a buildup of lactic acid that can result from too much of the drug building up in your body. Symptoms of lactic acidosis include:

- Tiredness
- Weakness
- Muscle aches
- Breathing difficulties
- Abdominal pain
- Dizziness
- Drowsiness

Precautions

Because of the increased risk of lactic acidosis, metformin usually isn't prescribed if you have kidney disease, liver disease, lung disease, heart failure or any other disease that may cause your body to produce too much lactic acid.

The following precautions also are important:

- If you drink alcohol daily or you occasionally overindulge, metformin and alcohol can produce lactic acidosis, making you sick. If you drink alcohol, discuss this with your doctor.
- If you take the gastrointestinal medication cimetidine (Tagamet), your dose of metformin may need to be lowered. Cimetidine can interfere with the ability of your kidneys to rid your body of metformin, causing a buildup of the drug and possible lactic acidosis.
- Because of the potential for lactic acidosis, it's important to stop taking metformin before having any procedure that involves the use of an intravenous (IV) dye. IV dyes are sometimes used in imaging procedures, such as a computerized tomography (CT) scan.

Alpha-glucosidase inhibitors

Alpha-glucosidase (AL-fuh-gloo-KOE-sih-days) inhibitors block the action of enzymes in the digestive tract that break down carbohydrates into glucose, delaying the digestion of carbohydrates. Glucose is absorbed into your bloodstream slower than usual, limiting the rapid rise in blood glucose that usually occurs right after a meal.

Two medications are in this class: acarbose (Precose) and miglitol (Glyset). You take them with each meal. Because these drugs aren't as effective as sulfonylureas or metformin in controlling blood glucose levels, they're typically prescribed along with other drugs to control high glucose levels after meals (postprandial elevations).

Possible side effects
Alpha-glucosidase inhibitors can cause gastrointestinal side effects, including abdominal bloating and pain, gas and diarrhea. These effects usually occur during the first few weeks and decrease with time. If you start with a low dose and gradually increase the amount, you're more likely to have mild instead of severe symptoms.

Used alone, these drugs don't cause hypoglycemia. But when taken with another oral diabetes medication, such as a sulfonylurea, or with insulin, you run a higher risk of low blood glucose. If you do experience hypoglycemia, drink milk or use glucose tablets or gel to treat it. Don't use table sugar (sucrose) or fruit juice because alpha-glucosidase inhibitors block the absorption.

Precautions
Because of possible digestive side effects, you shouldn't take acarbose or miglitol if you have these medical conditions:
- Irritable bowel syndrome
- Ulcerative colitis or Crohn's disease
- Partial intestinal obstruction or a predisposition for this problem
- A chronic malabsorption disorder, such as celiac disease
- Serious kidney or liver problems

If taken in high doses, acarbose can injure your liver. Fortunately, the damage is usually reversible by reducing the dose of the medication or discontinuing it.

Thiazolidinediones (TZDs)

Many people with type 2 diabetes have a resistance to insulin that prevents insulin from working properly. Thiazolidinediones (thi-uh-zole-uh-deen-DYE-owns), also called TZDs, help reduce blood glucose by making your body tissues more sensitive to insulin. The more effective insulin is at delivering glucose from your blood into your cells, the less glucose that remains in your bloodstream. This class of medications includes the drugs pioglitazone (Actos) and rosiglitazone (Avandia).

Possible side effects

Side effects from the medications may include swelling (edema) and weight gain from fluid retention. In some people who use TZDs, increased fluid retention leads to or worsens heart failure. Some of the following signs or symptoms could indicate heart failure. Contact your doctor right away if you experience:

- Shortness of breath
- Trouble sleeping, such as waking up short of breath
- Weakness or increased tiredness
- Rapid weight gain (from fluid retention)
- Swelling (edema) in your legs, ankles, feet

A rare but serious side effect of TZDs is liver injury. Before you take pioglitazone or rosiglitazone, your doctor should order blood tests to assess the health of your liver. It's also important to have your liver checked every two months during the first year of therapy. Contact your doctor right away if you experience signs and symptoms of liver damage, such as:

- Unexplained nausea
- Vomiting
- Abdominal pain
- Increased tiredness
- Loss of appetite
- Severe weight loss
- Dark urine
- Yellowing of your skin and eyes (jaundice)

Precautions

Taken alone, TZDs don't cause low blood glucose, but when used with a sulfonylurea or insulin, hypoglycemia can occur. TZDs may make birth control pills less effective. In addition, if you're a woman who's not ovulating but you haven't yet gone through menopause, it's possible that taking a TZD could cause you to start ovulating again, with risk of a pregnancy.

Meglitinides

Meglitinides (meh-GLIH-tin-ides) are chemically different from sulfonylureas, but their effects are similar. These medications cause a rapid, but short-lived, release of insulin by your pancreas. Because they work quickly and their effects wear off rapidly, the medications are taken with meals, kicking into action shortly after, when your blood glucose level is highest. Nateglinide (Starlix) and repaglinide (Prandin) are the only drugs in this class to receive Food and Drug Administration (FDA) approval. If you have liver or kidney disease, your doctor will typically take that into account in deciding if meglitinides are appropriate for you.

Possible side effects
Like sulfonylureas, meglitinides can cause low blood glucose (hypoglycemia). However, the risk of hypoglycemia is lower because of their short duration of action. These drugs may cause stomach upset in some people.

Precautions
If you miss a meal, skip that dose. Similar to sulfonylureas, be aware of possible drug interactions if you're taking other medications or using alcohol.

Oral drug combinations

The goal of combination therapy is to maximize the glucose-lowering effects of diabetes medications. By combining medications from different drug classes, the medications may work in two different ways to control your blood glucose. The most common combination therapy is to take two separate drugs at the same time. Two drugs also may be combined into one pill (see "Combination pills," page 132).

Some doctors prescribe three drugs at a time. More studies are necessary to determine the benefits of triple-drug therapy, but this may be an option if a combination of two oral medications doesn't achieve your goal.

A sulfonylurea and metformin

Sulfonylureas are often the base of combination therapy because of their ability to boost and maintain insulin secretion. A sulfonylurea combined with metformin is the most extensively studied drug combination. The medications seem to work more effectively together than they do individually. Metformin also is beneficial because it can help people who are overweight avoid additional weight gain and, in some cases, lose weight. Common side effects of this drug combination include nausea, diarrhea and a risk of low blood glucose.

A sulfonylurea and an alpha-glucosidase inhibitor

Combining acarbose or miglitol with a sulfonylurea is especially effective if you experience significant spikes in your blood glucose immediately after meals. Possible side effects include abdominal cramping, gas and diarrhea. You may also experience low blood glucose. Again, be sure to treat episodes of hypoglycemia with milk or glucose tablets or gel because alpha-glucosidase inhibitors block the absorption of table sugar and fruit juice.

Combination pills

Most combination therapies involve taking two separate drugs. However, the FDA has approved three types of combination pills:
- glipizide/metformin (Metaglip and generic)
- glyburide/metformin (Glucovance)
- rosiglitazone/metformin (Avandamet)

Although combination pills are convenient because you take fewer pills, there are trade-offs. For example, if you have a side effect, it's harder to tell which medication may be causing it. But if you took two separate pills, the doctor could advise cutting back on one at a time to see which one is linked with the side effect.

A sulfonylurea and a TZD

Adding a TZD medication to a sulfonylurea may help when the maximum dose of a sulfonylurea isn't working for you, you're overweight and your cells are highly insulin resistant. This combination also increases your risk of low blood glucose because TZDs improve your body's use of insulin stimulated by sulfonylureas.

Metformin and an alpha-glucosidase inhibitor

Studies consistently show that the combination of acarbose (an alpha-glucosidase inhibitor) and metformin is more effective in reducing blood glucose after meals than is metformin alone. Miglitol (another alpha-glucosidase inhibitor) hasn't been studied in combination with metformin as often as acarbose has been, but the same benefits are likely to apply.

Insulin

Insulin is generally associated with treatment of type 1 diabetes, but it's also an effective medication for treating type 2 diabetes. You may take insulin alone or you may use it in combination with an oral diabetes medication.

Your doctor may recommend insulin injections if you have poor control of your diabetes, because either your pancreas isn't making enough insulin or you aren't responding to other medications. Your doctor also may turn first to insulin if:

- Your fasting blood glucose level is markedly high — more than 300 mg/dL — and you have a high level of ketones in your urine
- You have a markedly high fasting blood glucose level and are experiencing symptoms of diabetes, such as excessive thirst and frequent urination
- You have gestational diabetes that can't be controlled by diet

You may need to take insulin for a short period to help bring your diabetes under control during an illness, or you may use the medication long term to keep your blood glucose in a safe range.

Possible side effects from combining metformin and an alpha-glucosidase inhibitor are the same as those associated with using metformin or an alpha-glucosidase inhibitor alone. Gastrointestinal symptoms are the most common side effect.

Metformin and a TZD

The TZDs pioglitazone and rosiglitazone are approved by the FDA for use with metformin. The combination therapy is more effective at reducing blood glucose than either class of medication alone. The precautions and side effects are the same as those listed for these drugs individually.

Oral drugs and insulin

Combining insulin with an oral medication can help both drugs work more effectively. The combination also can lower your daily insulin requirements and may limit weight gain associated with insulin therapy alone.

A sulfonylurea and insulin

Adding a dose of insulin at bedtime to your regular dosage of a sulfonylurea may improve blood glucose control. At first glance, a sulfonylurea and insulin don't appear to be a likely combination because they both boost insulin levels. However, they promote the circulation of insulin in different parts of your body. Using a sulfonylurea with insulin may allow you to use lower doses of insulin and achieve the same control. This treatment regimen is called bedtime insulin, daytime sulfonylurea (BIDS) therapy. BIDS therapy may be useful if a combination of a sulfonylurea and metformin hasn't worked for you.

Metformin and insulin

Similar to a sulfonylurea combination, combining metformin with insulin can reduce your insulin dose. Metformin helps your liver become more sensitive to insulin, making better use of it. Metformin also counteracts the problem of weight gain associated with insulin use. In fact, you may actually lose weight when using this combination. One theory is that metformin reduces appetite, causing you to consume fewer calories.

An alpha-glucosidase inhibitor and insulin

Acarbose, an alpha-glucosidase inhibitor, is approved by the FDA for use with insulin. Acarbose slows the absorption of carbohydrates, which may reduce your daily need for insulin, but this also increases risk of low blood glucose that can occur with insulin therapy. The alpha-glucosidase inhibitor miglitol hasn't been extensively studied in combination with insulin.

A TZD and insulin

This pairing is the most studied of the insulin combination therapies. If your blood glucose is well controlled, taking a TZD with insulin can reduce the amount of insulin you need each day. If you have trouble controlling your blood glucose, adding a TZD may help you better regulate your blood glucose levels. Side effects of this combination are low blood glucose and increased risk of fluid retention and heart failure in some people, along with the previously mentioned side effects of TZDs.

New injectable drugs

The FDA approved two new drugs in 2005: exenatide (Byetta) and pramlintide (Symlin). Both are injectable drugs. Exenatide may help prevent the need for insulin in people with type 2 diabetes. Pramlintide is used for better glucose control in addition to insulin in people with type 1 or type 2 diabetes.

Exenatide (Byetta)

If you can't control type 2 diabetes with oral drugs, you have another option before starting insulin. Exenatide (Byetta) is the first in a new class of drugs called incretin mimetics, which mimic the action of human hormones called incretins.

Exenatide comes in a pre-filled pen (needles aren't included). It's injected under the skin (subcutaneously) of your thigh, stomach area (abdomen) or upper arm before breakfast and evening meals.

Exenatide mimics the action of a hormone secreted by the gut — glucagon-like peptide-1 (GLP-1) — which prompts insulin production after a meal, but only if blood glucose levels are high. This action differs from current oral drugs, which promote insulin production regardless of blood glucose level. Exenatide also reduces the release of a hormone called glucagon, which would otherwise raise blood glucose after meals. Exenatide may also slow stomach emptying. These actions can greatly improve glucose control after meals.

Exenatide is used with metformin or a sulfonylurea, or a combination of metformin and a sulfonylurea. Exenatide may decrease your appetite, so you may eat less food, resulting in modest weight loss.

Side effects. The most common side effect of exenatide is nausea, which typically improves over time. Other common side effects include vomiting, diarrhea, dizziness, headache, feeling jittery and acid stomach. Exenatide taken along with a sulfonylurea increases the risk of hypoglycemia. The risk of hypoglycemia when using exenatide and a sulfonylurea may be lowered if the dose of sulfonylurea is reduced — talk with your doctor.

Pramlintide (Symlin)

The first in a new class of drugs called amylin mimetics, pramlintide (Symlin) mimics the action of the human hormone amylin, which is normally produced by the pancreas. Using a needle and syringe, you can inject pramlintide into your stomach area (abdomen) or your thigh immediately before meals. This slows down the movement of food through your stomach after meals. As a result, it affects how rapidly glucose enters your bloodstream. Pramlintide also appears to be linked with modest weight loss.

Pramlintide is designed for adults with type 1 or type 2 diabetes who require insulin and aren't reaching their target blood glucose levels. *Never* mix pramlintide and insulin in the same syringe.

Side effects. The most common side effect of pramlintide is nausea, which usually improves over time. Other potential side effects include vomiting, abdominal pain, headache, fatigue and dizziness. In addition, pramlintide is linked with an increased risk of insulin-induced severe hypoglycemia (seen within three hours of injecting pramlintide), particularly in people with type 1 diabetes. And severe hypoglycemia makes it difficult to think clearly, drive or do other activities. So follow your doctor's instructions carefully to reduce your risk of hypoglycemia. When you first start using pramlintide, your doctor will typically tell you to reduce your insulin amount by 50 percent.

Questions and answers

What should I do if I forget to take my medication?
That depends on which drugs you take. For example, alpha-glucosidase inhibitors should only be taken with meals. If you miss a dose, you may take it if you've just finished eating — otherwise, wait until the next meal. With certain drugs, such as metformin, if you're six or more hours late, don't take it, and don't double the next dose — just continue to follow your regular medication schedule. For specific recommendations, check the instructions that came with your prescription, or call your pharmacist or doctor for advice.

I heard there is a new drug for people with type 2 diabetes that helps control blood glucose and cholesterol. Is that true?
In 2005, an advisory committee of the FDA voted in favor of approving an oral drug called muraglitazar (Pargluva) for use in people with type 2 diabetes. This is the first in a new class of drugs that has two goals: to lower blood glucose and to improve blood fat levels (lower triglycerides and raise levels of HDL, the "good" cholesterol). This "two-in-one" pill would be convenient because many people with diabetes also have trouble controlling triglyceride and cholesterol levels. However, the FDA isn't bound by the advisory committee's recommendation. In addition, based on an analysis of five clinical trials, some cardiovascular experts have expressed major concerns about the incidence of serious adverse effects, including heart attack, stroke, heart failure, and even death. These experts are urging more extensive research before the drug is approved by the FDA.

Will any herbal remedies help treat type 2 diabetes?

Some people with diabetes do take herbal remedies in an effort to ease their symptoms, even though the effectiveness and side effects of these remedies are generally unknown. This is risky — manufacturers don't have to prove to the FDA that an herbal supplement is safe or effective before it goes on the market. And be very cautious about using herbal products manufactured or bought outside the United States. The American Diabetes Association cautions against the use of herbal supplements because little research exists to prove the remedies are safe and effective.

How can I keep my medication costs down?

Ask your doctor if your medication is available in a generic form, which usually costs less than a brand name. Also, ask your insurance provider if there's a list of drugs approved by your health plan, called a formulary. You'll pay more for drugs that aren't on that list. If you meet specific criteria, other options may include:

Medicare Part D. As of 2006, Medicare offers several drug benefit plans. Visit *www.medicare.gov* or call Medicare at (800) 633-4227.

Membership organizations. The AARP (formerly the American Association of Retired Persons) offers pharmacy services for members, often at a discount. Visit *www.aarp.org* or call (888) 687-2277. Also check for programs offered by professional organizations.

Patient assistance programs. Also called prescription assistance programs, these are for people who meet certain income and other requirements. To see if you qualify, call the Partnership for Prescription Assistance toll-free at (888) 477-2669 or visit *www.pparx.org*. Also visit NeedyMeds at *www.needymeds.com* or check the Web sites of drug companies. In addition, see the National Council on the Aging Web site at *www.ncoa.org* and click "BenefitsCheckUp."

State programs. Many states have programs to help people with low incomes pay for prescription drugs. Contact your state or local department of health or social services.

Military and veterans' benefits. Military personnel, veterans and their families may be eligible for the Tricare pharmacy program of the Department of Defense to save money on prescriptions. Visit *www.tricare.osd.mil/pharmacy* or call (877) 363-6337 toll-free.

Chapter 9

Dialysis and transplantation

G ood control of your blood sugar (glucose) levels and blood pressure are two key factors in helping to prevent kidney problems. Over several years, long-term kidney disease can lead to kidney failure, also called end-stage renal disease or ESRD, which is a serious, life-threatening condition. This is when your kidneys can no longer remove harmful wastes from your blood and your body retains extra fluid. (See "Kidney disease," page 33.)

Whether you have type 1 or type 2 diabetes, when your kidneys fail to work properly, you have two treatment options: kidney dialysis or a kidney transplant. Many people need dialysis while they're waiting for a kidney transplant. But there are other types of transplantation, including pancreas and islet cell transplants that attempt to restore insulin production in people with diabetes. The summaries in this chapter explain why these procedures are done and who may benefit from them.

The evaluation for any type of transplant will assess whether you:
- Are healthy enough to have surgery and tolerate lifelong post-transplant medications
- Have a medical condition that would make a transplant unlikely to succeed
- Are willing and able to take medications as directed
- Are strong enough emotionally to tolerate the typical long

wait for a donor organ and have family and friends who are supportive to help during this stressful time

Kidney dialysis

Kidney dialysis is an artificial means of removing waste products and extra fluid from your blood when your kidneys can no longer do this. There are two main types of dialysis: hemodialysis and peritoneal dialysis.

Hemodialysis

The most common form of dialysis is hemodialysis. It filters your blood through an artificial kidney (dialyzer) to remove extra fluids, chemicals and wastes. Blood is pumped out of your body to the artificial kidney through an access point (surgically created from your own blood vessels or a piece of tubing), usually in your arm. Surgery to make the access is usually done a couple of months before dialysis starts, to allow healing time.

Most people need treatment three times a week, about three to five hours at each session. This is usually done in a dialysis center, but it can be done at home if you have someone to help you. During dialysis, you may have side effects, such as unstable or low blood pressure, cramps or an upset stomach. Together with hemodialysis, medications (such as blood thinners, blood pressure medications and iron supplements) and a special diet will round out your treatment plan.

Peritoneal dialysis

This type of dialysis uses the network of tiny blood vessels in your abdomen (peritoneal cavity) to filter your blood. First, a surgeon implants a small, flexible tube (catheter) into your abdomen and allows healing time. Then you're ready to use one of the methods described below. With both methods, a dialysis solution is infused into and drained out of your abdomen to remove waste, chemicals and extra water. Each cycle is called an exchange. You can be more independent with peritoneal dialysis because you don't have to travel to a dialysis center.

Continuous ambulatory peritoneal dialysis (CAPD). CAPD can be done at home, work or any clean place — you perform the exchanges by hand instead of using a machine. Each exchange takes about 30 to 40 minutes, and it's done four or five times each day. Between exchanges, you can do your normal activities.

Continuous cycling peritoneal dialysis (CCPD). Also called automated peritoneal dialysis, a machine automatically infuses the cleansing fluid into your peritoneal cavity and drains it several times during the night while you sleep. This allows your days to be free, but you need to be attached to the machine at night for 10 to 12 hours.

Both CAPD and CCPD. If you weigh over 175 pounds or waste is filtered slowly, you may need a combination of CAPD and CCPD to get the right dialysis dose.

Drawbacks

Dialysis can dramatically change your lifestyle because of the frequent treatments needed. You'll also have to follow a special diet to manage your intake of protein, liquids, salt (sodium), potassium and phosphorus. If you use peritoneal dialysis, you must be careful about your technique to prevent serious abdominal infection that can start at the opening where the catheter enters your abdomen. In addition, many people on dialysis are prone to sleep disorders, bone problems, extra fluid buildup and other serious conditions.

A kidney transplant offers the best chance to restore normal kidney function and a more regular lifestyle. It also offers improved odds for long-term survival, but it's not without risks and there are long waiting lists.

Kidney transplant

A transplanted organ is a foreign tissue to your body. So a successful transplant depends on finding an organ that's a good match to minimize the chance that it will be rejected by your body. A successful transplant isn't a cure for kidney disease that's due to diabetes, but it usually restores sufficient kidney function and helps you feel better, so that you can become more active and have a better quality of life. It also frees you from dialysis.

Types of kidney transplants

To be considered for any type of transplant, the transplant center will register you on a nationwide waiting list. You may have a deceased-donor transplant or a living-donor transplant. Because few people sign up to be living donors, it's more common to get a kidney from a deceased donor.

The donor-recipient matching system considers blood type, tissue type and an antibody test (crossmatch), which determines whether the recipient has antibodies to the potential donor.

A transplant from a living donor has some advantages:

- If a donor is related by birth, you have a better chance of a good match.
- It's easier to evaluate the health of the donor and donor organ.

There's no need to put your name on the national waiting list if a close relative or friend intends to donate to you. Surgery can be scheduled in advance at an optimal time for donor and recipient, rather than being scheduled without advance notice upon the death of a donor.

Surgery and follow-up

The damaged kidney will most likely not be removed, and the surgeon will place the new kidney in your lower abdomen. The blood vessels of the new kidney will be attached to blood vessels in the lower part of your abdomen, just above one of your legs. The new kidney's ureter, the tube that links the kidney to the bladder, will be connected to your bladder.

Even with the best possible match between you and the donor, your immune system will try to reject the new kidney. Your drug regimen will include immunosuppressive drugs — drugs that suppress the activity of your immune system. You'll likely take these drugs for the rest of your life. These drugs may cause side effects, such as a round and full face, weight gain, acne, facial hair and stomach problems. These effects may decrease as time goes on.

Some immunosuppressive drugs can raise the risk of developing or worsening certain conditions, such as high blood pressure, high cholesterol and cancer. Because immunosuppressive drugs make your body more vulnerable to infection, your doctor may also prescribe antibacterial, antiviral and antifungal medications.

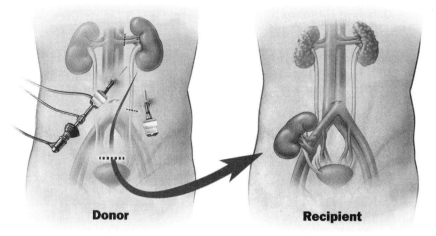

Donor   **Recipient**

In a minimally invasive living-donor kidney transplant, surgeons use small incisions to insert instruments to remove the donor kidney through an incision below the donor's bellybutton.

Your post-transplant treatment will be a delicate balancing act between preventing rejection and managing side effects, so your doctor will monitor your treatment closely.

Results

Results vary by the expertise and experience of the transplant center and other factors, such as the health and age of the candidate and the condition of the donated organ. From January 1988 through July 2005, there were more than 210,000 kidney transplants in the United States (but not all were diabetes-related), with about 71,400 from living donors.

The Organ Procurement and Transplantation Network provides these data on diabetes-related kidney transplants in the U.S. from 1997 through 2002:

- Living-donor transplants: About 97 percent of patients were living after one year and almost 87 percent after five years. The kidney was still functioning in almost 94 percent of patients after one year and almost 76 percent after five years.
- Deceased-donor transplants: When the organ was a close match, almost 96 percent of patients were living after one year and more than 80 percent after five years. The kidney was still functioning in more than 90 percent of patients after one year and more than 64 percent after five years. These statistics were

lower when the match wasn't as close (if criteria for organ donation were broader).

Survival rates are higher when the transplants are from living donors because the donor can be tested thoroughly for a good match, and living-donor kidneys typically last longer. With continuing advances, current statistics on kidney transplants may show even more favorable outcomes. (See "Results," page 146, for data on kidney-pancreas transplants.)

Pancreas transplant

A pancreas transplant is a treatment option if you have diabetes and are in kidney failure (also requiring a kidney transplant) or you don't respond well to standard insulin treatments. A successful pancreas transplant means insulin is no longer needed to control blood glucose, but it's far from a cure. There are life-threatening risks, especially if you have heart and blood vessel disease. The transplant center will evaluate you to see if you meet the eligibility requirements, including medical and emotional factors, similar to the criteria for a kidney transplant.

Types of pancreas transplants

Several different types of transplants involve the pancreas, as described below. Blood type, tissue type and an antibody test are key factors in the success of all types of pancreas transplants. Most pancreas transplants involve a whole pancreas from a deceased donor. The living-donor transplant procedure, in which a portion of the pancreas is donated, is still evolving.

Kidney-pancreas transplants. More than half of all pancreas transplants are performed at the same time as a kidney transplant. The strategy is to give you a healthy kidney and pancreas to reduce the potential for diabetes-related kidney damage in the future. In most cases, the organs come from the same deceased donor. This dual transplant appears to contribute to better survival rates for both organs.

Pancreas-after-kidney transplants. You may receive a pancreas transplant sometime after you've had a successful kidney transplant.

The treatment goal is similar to a kidney-pancreas transplant. The normal insulin function of your new pancreas should decrease the potential for diabetes-related kidney damage.

Pancreas-only transplants. Pancreas-only transplants (also called pancreas-alone transplants) are performed when there is normal or near-normal kidney function. Your doctor may recommend this option if you have frequent insulin reactions or poor blood glucose control despite the best efforts to manage your disease.

If your insulin treatment and other disease management strategies are working, a pancreas-only transplant is most likely not a better option. A study reported in 2003 indicated that people with working kidneys who received a pancreas-only transplant had significantly lower survival rates than those who used insulin and other conventional treatments. A pancreas that's transplanted along with a kidney is less likely to fail than a pancreas-only transplant.

Pancreas islet cell transplants. An experimental procedure called a pancreas islet cell transplant can provide new insulin-producing cells from a donor pancreas rather than a whole organ. As this minimally invasive procedure is improved, it may prove to be another viable option for people with type 1 diabetes. (See "Islet cell transplant," page 146.)

Surgery and follow-up

During surgery, your own pancreas will most likely not be removed. The surgeon will transplant the new pancreas with a small portion of the donor's small intestine still attached into your lower abdominal cavity. Your new pancreas should start working immediately, and your old pancreas will continue to perform its other functions.

Your immune system will try to reject the new pancreas, so your drug regimen will include immunosuppressive drugs. You'll likely take these drugs for the rest of your life. Some of these drugs may have major side effects, similar to those described under kidney transplant "Surgery and follow-up," page 142. The side effects of immunosuppressive drugs could be dangerous, and this must be weighed against the health problems caused by your diabetes.

Similar to a kidney transplant, your post-transplant treatment will be a balancing act between preventing rejection and managing side effects, with close monitoring by your doctor.

Results

As with kidney transplants, the results of pancreas transplants vary by the expertise and experience of the transplant center as well as factors such as the age and health of the candidate and the condition of the donated organ. From January 1988 through July 2005, there were more than 12,800 kidney-pancreas transplants and more than 4,500 pancreas transplants in the United States (but not all were diabetes-related). Almost all were from deceased donors, although in rare cases the patient received a portion of a pancreas from a living donor.

The Organ Procurement and Transplantation Network provides these data on diabetes-related pancreas transplants in the U.S. from 1995 to 2002:

- Kidney-pancreas transplants: Patient survival was almost 95 percent after one year and about 85 percent after five years. These organs were still functioning in about 92 percent of patients after one year and more than 75 percent of patients after five years.
- Pancreas-only transplants: Patient survival was more than 96 percent after one year and more than 80 percent after five years. The pancreas was still functioning in about 78 percent of patients after one year, but that dropped to about 47 percent after five years.

With continuing advances in pancreas transplantation, current statistics may show even more favorable outcomes.

Islet cell transplant

An experimental procedure called pancreas islet cell transplant shows much promise as a treatment option for some people with type 1 diabetes. With this transplant procedure, only the insulin-producing cells from a donor pancreas rather than the entire organ are transplanted into your body.

Throughout the pancreas are clusters of specialized cells, called the islets of Langerhans, which produce insulin. In type 1 diabetes, the body's immune system, which normally protects the body from viruses and bacteria, attacks and kills the islet cells.

An islet cell transplant has some of the same benefits as a pancreas transplant, but it's a less invasive surgery. However, there are still risks associated with this experimental procedure. As more people participate in clinical trials of this type of transplant, a clearer picture of its safety, long-term effects and potential as a treatment option will emerge.

How does an islet cell transplant work?

The procedure for an islet cell transplant continues to evolve, but most transplants follow the Edmonton Protocol — a method developed by several transplant centers and refined by the University of Alberta in Edmonton, Canada.

After a donor organ has been transferred to a transplant center, lab technicians extract only the islet cells and purify them. Then a specialist called an interventional radiologist performs the islet cell transplant. Using image-guided methods, the radiologist directs a tube through an opening in your abdomen to the portal vein, a blood vessel leading into your liver. The islet cells are transplanted through this tube to your liver. The cells spread throughout the liver, attaching to small blood vessels. The liver is a good site for the transplant because it's easier to get to than your pancreas, and the islet cells seem to do well in that location.

About a million islets are needed for a transplant to be effective in an average-sized person. Usually two or more donor organs are necessary to get enough islets for a single transplant. As donor organs become available, there are more cell infusions until the desired insulin production is reached.

Your body will regard the new cells as it would a new organ — foreign tissue. So a successful transplant depends on a treatment regimen that includes immunosuppressive drugs, which can have serious side effects, as discussed earlier in this chapter. In addition, the availability of islet cells is very limited because of the shortage of organ donors.

How effective are islet cell transplants?

Of the 267 transplants performed worldwide from 1990 to 1999, only 8 percent of the people receiving them were free of insulin treatments one year after the transplant. The new Edmonton Protocol improved greatly on these outcomes, mainly by increasing the number of transplanted cells and modifying the number and doses of immunosuppressive drugs. But information about success rates is limited.

In 2001, the National Institute of Diabetes and Digestive and Kidney Diseases established the Collaborative Islet Transplant Registry (CITR) to collect and analyze data on islet cell transplants performed at centers in the United States and Canada. The CITR's 2005 annual report presented data on 138 patients. At one year after patients' final infusions, 58 percent no longer needed insulin. Those who still needed insulin treatment after one year experienced an average reduction of 69 percent of their daily insulin requirements.

Choosing a transplant center

You'll need a doctor's referral to get an evaluation by a transplant center to see if you're a good candidate. The United Network for Organ Sharing (UNOS) Web site at *www.transplantliving.org* can guide you in making decisions about a transplant center. It also includes information on financial resources, the transplant process, medications and more. You can also call UNOS Patient Services' toll-free number at (888) 894-6361. Carefully consider important issues, such as:

- Which transplant centers are covered under your insurance plan? What portion will you need to pay? Is financial aid available, or can they help you check out other funding sources?
- How many transplants (of the type you're seeking) does the center perform each year?
- What are the organ and patient survival rates? Compare transplant center data maintained by the Scientific Registry of Transplant Recipients: Visit *www.ustransplant.org* and look for "Center-Specific Reports." Find your state, the type of transplant,

and then centers within your state for details such as number of transplants performed, waiting time and patient outcomes.

- What other services does the center provide? Many centers assist you with travel arrangements, help you find local housing for your recovery period or direct you to organizations that can help with these concerns.

If the transplant center medical team determines that you're a good candidate, and a relative or close friend wants to donate an organ to you, the transplant center handles the matching and the surgery process. Otherwise the transplant center will register you on a nationwide waiting list maintained by UNOS. UNOS matches donors to recipients.

The wait can be long — several factors are involved, such as your medical status, the condition of the donated organ, how close you live to the available organ, and how long you've been on the waiting list. Your transplant center will notify you when an organ is available.

Questions and answers

Are there any studies looking at ways to eliminate the need for the lifelong use of immunosuppressive drugs following a transplant?

Yes. A number of research centers throughout the world are investigating tolerogenic (tol-uh-ro-JEN-ik) drugs. These newer and less potent medications would trick your body into accepting the transplanted cells and organs. The drugs work by shutting off a small part of your immune system — just enough to keep the new cells from being attacked. If the medications work, you would no longer need to take immunosuppressive drugs indefinitely.

Can islet cells be transplanted into a child with newly diagnosed type 1 diabetes?

That's the long-term goal of researchers — to catch the disease early and eliminate it before it has a chance to do any damage. Until recently, islet cell transplantation would never have been considered for a child, let alone most adults, with type 1 diabetes.

This thinking could possibly change if current research efforts are successful. Presently, though, only adults with type 1 diabetes are considered appropriate candidates for islet cell transplantation.

How do I find out more about participating in clinical trials for islet cell transplantation?

Ask your doctor if you might be an appropriate candidate and how to find out about clinical trials. The criteria will likely include a certain age range, weight range, a minimum number of years with type 1 diabetes, a certain degree of disease severity, good general health and evidence of careful disease management. You also can search a Web site maintained by the National Institutes of Health at *www.clinicaltrials.gov* and search for "islet cell transplant." Contact the American Diabetes Association to learn more about islet cell transplantation research and its progress. (See "Additional resources," page 219.)

Part 4

Successful management

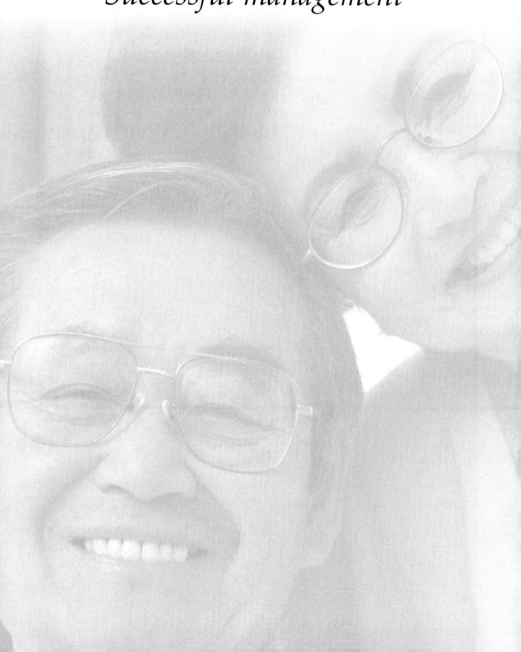

Chapter 10

Important tests:
Are you getting them?

Within weeks to months after your diagnosis, managing your diabetes should start to become routine. You'll gradually develop a pattern for testing your blood sugar (glucose), exercising and eating. But you often may wonder, "How am I doing?" You'd like to know if your daily efforts at controlling your blood glucose are paying off and keeping other health problems at bay.

You can find out the answer by keeping in regular contact with your health care team and making sure you receive appropriate tests during your checkups. These tests can assess how well you're doing in controlling your blood glucose and spot potential problems.

Regular checkups are important because they:
- Provide your doctor with an opportunity to check for early stages of diabetes complications. Many potential complications show up early in simple blood and urine tests and exams done in your doctor's office.
- Allow you and your doctor to review your successes and difficulties at meeting your blood glucose goals.
- Give you an opportunity to hear suggestions from members of your health care team on how to meet your goals.

Your health care team

Successful management of diabetes usually involves working with several professionals. Your health care team may include the following:

Primary doctor. Look for a doctor who specializes in diabetes, such as a board-certified endocrinologist.

Nurse. A nurse, preferably a certified diabetes educator (explained below), can help you learn more about your diabetes and counsel you on self-care.

Registered dietitian. A registered dietitian can work with you to develop a healthy-eating plan to help control your blood glucose levels.

Eye doctor. An eye doctor (ophthalmologist or optometrist) who has expertise in diabetes-related eye problems can help detect early eye disease.

Foot doctor. A foot doctor (podiatrist) who has expertise in diabetes-related foot problems can detect and treat foot problems, such as calluses or sores, and help you learn how to prevent future problems.

Other professionals. Depending on your needs, you may also benefit from seeing other professionals, such as a nephrologist (kidney specialist), neurologist (nerve specialist) or a mental health professional. Look for professionals who have experience and expertise in working with people who have diabetes.

What is a certified diabetes educator?

A certified diabetes educator (CDE) is a professional who has passed a national exam on diabetes education and is certified to teach people with diabetes how to manage their disease. Although a CDE is often a registered nurse or a registered dietitian, other professionals, such as physicians, physician assistants and pharmacists, also may be certified.

How often you should see your doctor or other members of your health care team depends on what's happening with your health. If you're having trouble keeping your blood glucose levels down or if you're changing medication, you may need to contact a member of your health care team weekly. Your doctor may even recommend that you check in more often until your blood glucose and insulin doses stabilize.

In general, though, if you're feeling good and keeping your blood glucose within the range that you and your doctor have agreed upon, you probably won't need to see your doctor more than four times a year — about once every three months. If you reach and are able to maintain your blood glucose goals, the visits may be less often.

What to expect during a checkup

Your doctor will likely begin your exam by asking you questions about your blood glucose readings and overall health: How have you been feeling? Have you been experiencing any new symptoms or problems? Have you been able to keep your blood glucose within your target range? It's important to bring your daily log of blood glucose readings with you to your appointment so that your doctor can review it. Any episodes of high or low blood glucose need to be discussed to try to determine what caused them.

Other issues your doctor may want to cover include:

- Temporary adjustments you made to your treatment program, including changes in medication, to accommodate for high or low blood glucose readings
- Problems you may be having in following your treatment program
- Emotional and social problems you may be experiencing
- Changes in your use of tobacco or alcohol

During your checkup, a member of your health care team typically will also:

Check your blood pressure. High blood pressure (hypertension) can damage your blood vessels, and you're already at increased risk of blood vessel disease if you have diabetes. Diabetes and high blood pressure are often associated, and when teamed together they significantly increase your risk of a heart attack or stroke. If your blood pressure is high, you may need to take medication to control it. Controlling your high blood pressure can help prevent diabetes complications. (See "Monitor your blood pressure," page 175.)

Check your weight. If you have diabetes and you're overweight or obese, losing weight can help you control your blood glucose — gaining more weight will make it harder to manage your glucose. If you take a diabetes medication, weight loss may reduce your need for medication.

Check your feet. At each visit you should have a brief examination of your feet. At least once a year you should have a thorough foot exam. During a thorough exam, here's what your doctor is looking for:

- Breaks in the skin, which could lead to an infection
- Foot pulses, which indicate if you have good blood circulation in the foot, and a sense of touch, which indicates if sensory nerves in the foot are working properly
- Normal range of motion, to make sure there is no muscle or bone damage
- Bony deformations or evidence of increased pressure, such as calluses, which may indicate that you need different shoes

If a problem is identified, examine your feet regularly to make sure the condition doesn't worsen. If you're unable to examine your feet yourself, recruit the help of a family member or a close friend.

Request blood and urine tests. Simple blood and urine tests can detect early signs of diabetes complications, such as kidney disease. The earlier you discover and treat emerging problems, the better your chances of stopping, or at least slowing, the damage.

The following four tests are especially important. Three of them examine your blood and one checks your urine.

A1C test

An A1C test, also known as a glycated hemoglobin test, is an effective tool for determining how well you're managing your blood glucose. This blood test is different from a fasting blood glucose test or a daily finger stick, both of which only measure your blood glucose at any given moment. An A1C test indicates your average blood glucose level over the past two to three months. Here's how that works:

Some of the glucose in your bloodstream attaches to hemoglobin, a protein found in red blood cells. This is known as glycated hemoglobin or A1C.

To check your A1C level, blood is usually drawn from a vein in your arm, and the sample is sent to a lab for analysis. Although some home test kits are available, it's important that this test be done correctly. Test results indicate what percentage of your hemoglobin is glycated (sugar coated):

- 4 percent to 6 percent is normal for people without diabetes
- Less than 7 percent is the typical goal for most people with diabetes
- More than 7 percent is a concern and may indicate a need for a change in your treatment plan

Talk with your doctor to find out your specific goal. Although an A1C level under 7 percent is a common target, your doctor may recommend a level under 6 percent if you're pregnant or you need a stricter goal for other reasons.

The normal range for A1C values may vary somewhat among labs across the country. If you've had testing done elsewhere and you're seeing a new doctor, it's important that your doctor take this possible variation into account when interpreting your test results.

How often should I have it done?

If your therapy has recently changed or you're not meeting your blood glucose goals, your doctor will likely recommend an A1C test every three months. If you're able to control your blood glucose levels and meet treatment goals, an A1C test is recommended at least twice a year.

How does it help?

An A1C test can help in many ways. Say for instance you're having trouble maintaining a normal blood glucose level and your doctor is deciding whether to prescribe medication or allow more time for

Exams, tests and quick checks

If you have diabetes, you'll need regular exams and tests to watch for current or potential health problems. Test results may indicate a need to change your treatment plan.

Which ones	How often
Blood pressure check*	At every visit with your doctor
Weight check	At every visit with your doctor
Foot exam*	Brief check at every visit with your doctor; thorough exam at least once a year
Eye exam*	At least once a year, but more often if you have eye problems, poorly controlled diabetes, high blood pressure, kidney disease, or you're pregnant
A1C test (glycated hemoglobin test)	At least two times a year if you're meeting treatment goals and blood glucose is stable; about every three months if you're not meeting glucose goals or your treatment changed
Lipid panel (cholesterol and triglyceride levels*)	At least once a year, but more often if needed to achieve your goals; every two years if lipid values are at low-risk levels (LDL less than 100 mg/dL, HDL over 50 mg/dL, triglycerides under 150 mg/dL)
Serum creatinine test	Once a year, but more often if you have kidney disease or are taking medications that could have a harmful effect on your kidneys
Urine test for protein (urine microalbumin test)	Once a year, starting five years after the diagnosis of type 1 diabetes, or starting when type 2 diabetes is diagnosed (also recommended during pregnancy for women with diabetes)

*See Chapter 11 for more details.

you to improve your diet and exercise plan. Your doctor may have you increase the amount of time you exercise for two or three months and then have you come in for another A1C test. If the test shows an improved reading, then increased exercise may be all that you need to control your blood glucose, and your doctor may not prescribe medication.

In addition, the test is a way to alert you and your doctor to potential problems. If you've had normal A1C readings for several months or years and suddenly you have an abnormal reading, this may be a sign that your treatment plan needs a change, including more frequent blood glucose testing. Results of the A1C test also indicate your risk of complications from diabetes — the higher your test result is, the greater your risk.

Lipid panel

A lipid panel measures the fats (lipids) in your blood, including cholesterol and triglycerides. Blood is drawn from a vein in your arm and sent to a lab. To get an accurate reading, it's best to fast for nine to 12 hours before blood is drawn.

The measurements can indicate your risk of having a heart attack or other heart disease. The panel typically includes:

Low-density lipoprotein (LDL) cholesterol. This "bad" cholesterol promotes accumulation of fatty deposits (plaques) in your arteries. These plaques choke off blood supply to the heart and other vital organs.

High-density lipoprotein (HDL) cholesterol. This "good" cholesterol protects against heart disease by helping clear excess cholesterol from your body. This keeps your arteries open and your blood circulating more freely.

Triglycerides. A normal amount of these blood fats is needed for good health to help your body store fat that's later used for energy. But high levels of triglycerides increase your risk of heart and blood vessel disease.

Total cholesterol. This is the sum of your blood's LDL cholesterol, HDL cholesterol and a portion of triglycerides. Higher levels may put you at greater risk of heart and blood vessel disease.

How often should I have it done?

People who don't have diabetes need a lipid panel at least every five years — more often if their blood fat levels are above normal or they have a family history of elevated blood fats. If you have diabetes, you'll need a lipid panel at least once a year, but more often if you're not achieving your lipid goals. If your lipid values are at low-risk levels (LDL less than 100 mg/dL, HDL over 50 mg/dL, triglycerides under 150 mg/dL) a lipid panel every two years may be enough. However, if you have cardiovascular disease, your doctor may recommend a goal of less than 70 mg/dL for LDL cholesterol with the use of a cholesterol-lowering drug called a statin. (For target lipid goals for people with diabetes, see "Know your ABCs," page 176.)

How does it help?

A rising level of blood fats can alert your doctor to increased risk of blood vessel damage. That's because diabetes can accelerate the development of clogged and hardened arteries (atherosclerosis), which increases your risk of a heart attack, stroke and poor circulation in your feet and legs. Knowing your blood fat levels also helps your doctor determine if you could benefit from medication to lower your cholesterol or triglyceride levels. Diet and exercise are the first defenses against unhealthy blood fat levels, just as they are in managing diabetes. Your doctor may prescribe lipid-lowering medication if these steps aren't effective or if your LDL or triglyceride levels are above your target goals.

Serum creatinine test

A serum creatinine (kree-AT-ih-nin) test measures the level of creatinine in your blood and can alert you and your doctors to kidney problems. Creatinine is a waste byproduct of creatine, a protein that supplies energy for muscle contraction.

Your blood normally produces a small but relatively constant amount of creatinine. If the creatinine level in your blood rises above normal, it's a sign that your kidneys have been damaged and aren't able to function properly (renal insufficiency). The higher the creatinine level, the more advanced the kidney disease.

Normal values of serum creatinine vary, depending on your sex, muscle mass and other factors, so ask your doctor what's normal for you. Different labs may have slightly different normal ranges. At Mayo Clinic, normal ranges are:

- 0.9 to 1.4 mg/dL for men
- 0.7 to 1.2 mg/dL for women

How often should I have it done?

You should have a serum creatinine test once a year. If you have known kidney damage, or you're taking medications that could have a harmful effect on your kidneys, your doctor may recommend that you have this test more often.

How does it help?

Knowing the health of your kidneys is important because kidney function influences many decisions regarding your medical care, including which medications are safe for you to take and how aggressive to be in controlling your blood pressure.

Urine test for protein

A urine test that detects tiny (microscopic) amounts of protein (albumin), called a microalbumin test, also is used to assess the health of your kidneys. When your kidneys are functioning normally, they filter out wastes in your blood, and these wastes are removed through urination. Protein and other helpful substances remain in the bloodstream. When your kidneys become damaged, the opposite occurs — waste products remain in your blood and protein leaks into your urine.

The preferred method to screen for protein leakage is the spot collection, using about the same amount of urine provided during routine urine testing (urinalysis). This easy collection, done at a medical visit, generally provides accurate information. An alternative but cumbersome method is to save all of your urine over a 24-hour period in a jug that you get from your doctor. You then return the urine jug to your doctor's office, where it's sent to a lab and analyzed.

When your kidneys first begin to leak, typically only tiny amounts of protein escape. In the early stage of kidney disease, you may have a condition called microalbuminuria (mi-kro-al-bu-min-U-ree-uh). A more advanced stage of the disease, called macroalbuminuria or clinical albuminuria, can occur after you've had diabetes for many years.

Typically, here's what your urine test results will mean, measured as milligrams (mg) of protein leakage:

- Less than 30 mg is normal
- 30 to 299 mg indicates early stage of kidney disease (microalbuminuria)
- 300 mg or more indicates advanced kidney disease (macroalbuminuria)

Protein in the urine can occur for reasons other than diabetes, so if your test results are higher than normal, you may be tested again at another time to confirm that you have kidney disease.

Urine testing at home

Different types of home urine test kits are available, but they vary in quality — and some types aren't reliable. Depending on the kit, you can test for:

- Glucose
- Ketones
- Glucose and ketones
- Microscopic amounts of protein (microalbuminuria)

Glucose kits, available in strip form, aren't recommended because they're much less reliable than results obtained from blood glucose meters. Ketone kits, also available in strip form, detect some ketones, but not all of them. So these kits are less reliable than blood ketone testing meters, but they're still helpful and often recommended. Ketone test strips reveal results through color changes. Some doctors recommend both ketone testing meters and home test kits to check for ketones.

With a kit that checks for microalbuminuria, you mail a urine sample to a lab. A doctor must interpret the results. Ask your doctor for more information.

How often should I have it done?

You should have a urine test for protein (microalbumin test) once a year, starting five years after the diagnosis of type 1 diabetes or starting when type 2 diabetes is diagnosed. The test is also recommended during pregnancy for women with diabetes.

How does it help?

A urine test for protein can alert you and your doctor to kidney damage — it's essential to identify this in an early stage.

By keeping your blood glucose level within a normal or near-normal range, you can help prevent the progression of kidney disease. Controlling high blood pressure also is important in preventing further kidney damage. Blood pressure medications called angiotensin-converting enzyme (ACE) inhibitors often are prescribed to people with kidney damage because they help protect kidney function. Other classes of blood pressure drugs also can be beneficial, and you may need more than one type.

Eating a low-protein diet may improve protein leakage by reducing the workload on your kidneys. The typical American diet is high in protein — your diabetes educator can give you advice on a low-protein diet if you need one.

Questions and answers

Will exercising heavily or changing my diet a few days before an A1C test affect the results?

You can't alter the findings by changing your diet or exercise routine a few days before the test. You can get an inaccurate reading, however, if you've had a recent blood transfusion or you've experienced certain types of anemia.

If one A1C test result is above my goal, should my treatment plan be changed? Or is it better to see if future tests results are also above normal?

One test above your goal is definitely sufficient reason to reassess your treatment plan, because this test indicates how well you've controlled your blood glucose during the past two to three months.

But this doesn't mean that your program needs to be completely changed. Your doctor may recommend that you monitor your blood glucose more often, watch your diet more closely, get more physical activity or make dosage adjustments to your medications.

How much weight do I have to lose to improve my lipid levels?
Losing as little as 5 percent to 10 percent of your weight can lower your triglycerides, raise your HDL ("good") cholesterol level and possibly lower your LDL ("bad") cholesterol level. Greater weight loss may bring even more improvement.

What should I do if I feel that I'm not getting adequate follow-up care from my doctor?
Discuss your concerns regarding your treatment with your doctor. In areas where you're having problems, ask for suggestions on how to remedy them. If your primary care doctor isn't able to provide you with the information you need, ask to see another health professional who likely can: a doctor who's a diabetes specialist (endocrinologist), a nurse who's a certified diabetes educator, a registered dietitian, or one of the other professionals listed under "Your health care team," page 154. You should feel comfortable with the care you're receiving and have open communication with your health care team.

Chapter 11

Self-care: Reducing your risk of complications

T reating your diabetes isn't a job that you can delegate solely to your doctor. It takes teamwork. Your health care team can provide helpful advice, information and care, but it's up to you to follow through. You're in the driver's seat.

It's also important that you approach your disease proactively instead of reactively. You want to prevent complications rather than simply respond to them when they occur. So take the following steps to help improve your chances for a smooth ride ahead.

Have a yearly physical

Beyond your regular checkups to monitor your diabetes treatment, once a year have a thorough physical exam. An annual physical is an opportunity to screen for conditions such as kidney or heart disease, which may not be part of your regular diabetes checkups. In addition, you may be so focused on your diabetes that you don't notice signs and symptoms associated with another condition. During an annual physical these features may come to light.

If you have a family or primary care doctor, he or she can perform the physical exam. Your diabetes specialist also may serve as your primary care doctor, particularly if you have type 1 diabetes.

> ### Medicare: Diabetes Self-Management Training
>
> If you have Medicare Part B, you may be eligible for coverage for Diabetes Self-Management Training. This training includes how to manage your blood glucose, lifestyle issues, and preventing and treating complications of diabetes. If you meet certain criteria, Medicare helps cover 10 hours of initial training in a Medicare-approved program during a 12-month period, plus two hours of follow-up each year.
>
> This service requires a prescription. Ask your doctor or diabetes educator if you're a candidate. Out-of-pocket expenses will depend on which Medicare plan you're enrolled in.

Get a yearly eye exam

Diabetes is the leading cause of new cases of blindness in people ages 20 to 74. The American Diabetes Association (ADA) recommends an initial comprehensive eye exam by an eye specialist (ophthalmologist or optometrist) shortly after diagnosis if you have type 2 diabetes and within five years after onset if you have type 1 diabetes. After that, have an eye exam by a specialist yearly, or more often if you have eye damage (retinopathy) that's getting worse.

If your diabetes is poorly controlled, you have high blood pressure or kidney disease, or you are pregnant, you may need to see an eye specialist more than once a year. If your eyes are normal after an exam and your blood sugar (glucose) is under control, your eye specialist may recommend an eye exam every two to three years. But don't wait for vision problems to develop before you see an eye specialist. Typically, by the time symptoms emerge, some permanent damage has already occurred.

Choose an eye specialist who has expertise and experience in diabetic retinopathy. Make sure this person knows you have diabetes and performs a thorough exam, including dilation of your pupils. This exam generally includes the following:

Visual acuity test. A visual acuity test determines your level of vision and need for corrective lenses, and it establishes a baseline measurement for future exams.

External eye exam. An external eye exam measures your eye movements, along with the size of your pupils and their ability to respond to light.

Retinal exam. When doing a retinal exam, your eye specialist places medicated eyedrops into your eyes to dilate your pupils and check for damage to your retinas and the tiny blood vessels that nourish them. This is an especially important test because retinal damage is the most common eye complication of diabetes.

Glaucoma test. A glaucoma test (tonometry) measures the pressure in your eyes, which helps detect glaucoma, a disease that can gradually narrow your field of vision and produce tunnel vision and blindness. Diabetes increases your risk of developing glaucoma.

Slit-lamp exam. During a slit-lamp exam, your eye specialist evaluates the structures of your eyes, such as the cornea and iris. He or she also looks for cataracts, which cloud your lenses and can make you feel as if you're looking through wax paper or a smudgy window. Diabetes can spur cataracts to develop sooner than they otherwise would.

Eye photography. If you have eye damage or suspected damage, photos may be taken with specially designed cameras to document the status of your vision and establish a baseline for future exams.

See your dentist regularly

High blood glucose can impair your immune system, making it difficult to fight off bacteria and viruses that cause infection.

One common site of infection is your gums. That's because your mouth harbors many bacteria. If these germs settle in your gums and cause an infection, you may end up with gum disease that can cause your teeth to loosen and fall out.

In addition, limited research suggests that people with gum infections may be at increased risk of cardiovascular disease. One theory is that bacteria from the mouth gets into the bloodstream and may cause inflammation throughout the body, including the arteries. This may be linked with the development of artery-clogging plaques, possibly increasing the risk of a heart attack or stroke.

To help prevent damage to your gums and teeth:
- See your dentist twice a year, and make sure your dentist knows that you have diabetes.
- Brush your teeth twice a day, using a soft nylon toothbrush, and brush the upper surface of your tongue.
- Floss every day.
- Look for early signs of gum disease, such as bleeding gums, redness and swelling. If you notice them, see your dentist.

Keep up-to-date on your vaccinations

Because high blood glucose can weaken your immune system, you may be more prone to complications from influenza and pneumonia than people who don't have diabetes — if you have heart or kidney disease, you're at even higher risk.

Annual flu shot

The best way to avoid the flu (influenza) or to reduce its symptoms is to have an annual flu shot (vaccination). In the United States, the best time to be vaccinated is in October or November. This allows your immunity to peak during the height of the flu season, which is generally December through March. But in other parts of the world, the flu season varies: In the Southern Hemisphere it's primarily from April to September, and in the tropics you can catch the flu year-round. So take this into account if you're traveling and get advice from your doctor or a travel medicine specialist.

In the United States, flu shots are modified annually to protect you against those flu strains most likely to circulate during the coming winter. The vaccine contains only noninfectious viruses and can't cause the flu. The most common side effect is a little soreness at the spot where the injection is given. Ask your doctor if there are any other risks in your case.

Pneumonia vaccine

Most doctors recommend that people with diabetes receive the pneumonia (pneumococcal) vaccine. For healthy people age 65 or older, generally just one lifetime dose is recommended unless they were younger than 65 when first vaccinated. However, a one-time booster dose after five years is often recommended if you have diabetes, renal failure or kidney transplantation. Check with your doctor for advice.

The pneumonia vaccine contains antigens — substances that activate your immune system — that protect you against 85 percent to 90 percent of all forms of pneumonia found in the United States. Side effects of the pneumococcal vaccine are generally minor and include mild soreness or swelling at the injection site.

Others

Make sure you're up-to-date on other important immunizations, such as a tetanus shot and a booster shot every 10 years. Ask your doctor about getting vaccinated for protection against hepatitis B if you receive hemodialysis.

Care for your feet

Diabetes can cause two potentially dangerous threats to your feet: It can damage the nerves in your feet, and it can reduce blood flow to your feet. When the network of nerves in your feet is damaged, the sensation of pain in your feet is reduced. Because of this, you can develop a blister or cut your foot without realizing it. Diabetes also can narrow your arteries, reducing blood flow to your feet. With less blood to nourish tissues in your feet, it's harder for sores to heal. An unnoticed cut or sore hidden beneath your socks and shoes can quickly develop into a larger problem.

Do you have PAD?

If you experience a burning or aching pain in your feet or toes when you're resting, or have a leg or foot sore that doesn't heal, you may have severe peripheral arterial disease (PAD). The first symptoms of PAD may be leg pain or cramping when walking, which disappears with rest. Talk with your doctor if you have these signs or symptoms. PAD is a major risk factor for amputation of lower limbs. And people with PAD have a greater risk of heart attack and stroke. (See "Peripheral arterial disease," page 31.)

Check your feet every day

Use your eyes and hands to examine your feet. If you can't see some parts of your feet, use a mirror or ask a family member or a friend to examine those locations. Look for the following:

- Blisters, cuts and bruises
- Cracking, peeling and wrinkling
- Redness, red streaks and swelling
- Feet that are pinker, paler, darker or redder than usual, possibly due to pressure from tight shoes

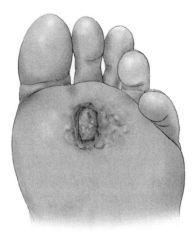

Diabetes can impair blood flow to your feet and cause nerve damage. Without proper attention and care, a small injury can develop into an open sore (ulcer) that can be difficult to treat.

Keep your feet clean and dry

Wash your feet each day with lukewarm water. To avoid burning your feet, test the water temperature with a thermometer. It should be no warmer than 90 F (32 C). Or test the water by touching a dampened washcloth to a sensitive area of your body, such as your face, neck or wrist.

Wash your feet with a gentle, massage-like motion, using a soft washcloth or sponge and a mild soap. Dry your skin by blotting or patting. Don't rub because you may accidentally damage your skin. Dry carefully between your toes to help prevent fungal infection.

Moisturize your skin

When diabetes damages your nerves, you may sweat less than normal, leaving your skin dry, especially on your feet. Dry skin can itch and crack, increasing your risk of an infection. To prevent dry skin, use a moisturizer regularly.

Keep the blood flowing

To help keep blood flowing to your feet, put your feet up when sitting, then move your ankles and toes frequently. Don't cross your legs for long and don't wear tight socks.

Wear clean, dry socks

Wear socks made of fibers that pull (wick) sweat away from your skin, such as cotton and special acrylic fibers — not nylon. Avoid those with tight elastic bands that reduce circulation or that are thick or bulky. Bulky socks often fit poorly, and a poor fit can irritate your skin. It's also a good idea to avoid mended socks with thick seams that can rub and irritate your skin. Indentations from the seams in socks aren't a problem for most people, but among people with diabetes they can cause pressure sores.

Trim your toenails carefully

Cut your toenails straight across so that they are even with the end of your toe. File rough edges so that you don't have any sharp areas that could cut the neighboring toe. Be especially careful not to injure the surrounding skin. If you notice redness around the nails, report this to your regular doctor or your podiatrist.

Use foot products cautiously

Don't use a file or scissors on calluses, corns or bunions. You can injure your feet that way. Also, don't put chemicals on your feet, such as wart removers. See your regular doctor or podiatrist for problem calluses, corns, bunions or warts.

Wear shoes to protect your feet from injury

To help prevent injury to your feet and toes:

Protect against heat and cold. Don't use heating pads on your feet. Use proper footwear to avoid hot pavement in hot weather and to avoid frostbite in cold weather.

Always wear shoes. Around the house wear sturdy slippers.

Check your shoes. Look inside your shoes for tears or rough edges that might injure your feet. Shake out your shoes before you put them on to make sure nothing is inside, such as a pebble.

Select a comfortable and safe style of shoe. Good shoe design includes:

- *Soft leather tops.* Leather adapts to the shape of your foot and lets air circulate. Good air circulation reduces sweating, a major cause of skin irritation.

- *Closed-toe design.* Shoes with closed toes provide the best protection.
- *Low-heeled shoes.* These shoes are safer, more comfortable and less damaging to your feet.
- *Flexible soles made from crepe or foam rubber.* These soles are most comfortable for daily wear. They also act as good shock absorbers. Soles should provide solid footing and not be slippery.

Have at least two pairs of shoes so that you can switch shoes each day. This gives your shoes time to completely dry out and regain their shape. Don't wear wet shoes because moisture can shrink the material and make your shoes rub against your feet.

When to see your doctor

Consider taking your shoes and socks off every time you visit your doctor to make sure your doctor examines your feet routinely. Keep in mind that even people who take good care of their feet sometimes develop foot sores. Most of these should begin to heal within a couple of days to two weeks. However, if a wound isn't healing, appears to be getting bigger or looks as if it may be infected, see your regular doctor or a foot care doctor (podiatrist).

Also see your doctor if you have a tingling feeling, numbness or pain in your feet or toes. This could indicate nerve damage. (See "Nerve damage," page 32.)

Consulting a podiatrist

Because foot care is especially important to people with diabetes, your primary care doctor or diabetes specialist may recommend a podiatrist — a doctor who specializes in foot care. A podiatrist can teach you how to trim your toenails properly. If you have vision problems or significant loss of sensation in your feet, he or she can trim them for you.

A podiatrist also can teach you how to buy properly fitted shoes and prevent problems such as corns and calluses. If problems do occur, a podiatrist can help treat them to prevent more serious conditions from developing. Even small sores can quickly turn into serious problems without proper treatment.

Does the shoe fit?

When you buy new shoes:

- Make sure the tip of each shoe extends at least a quarter inch beyond your longest toe. The shoe tip also should be wide and long enough that your toes aren't cramped. Walk around the store with both of the new shoes on.
- If possible, try on shoes in early afternoon. Feet swell as the day goes on. If you buy shoes in the morning, they may feel too tight later on. Getting fitted at the end of the day may give you a fit that's too roomy in the morning.
- If one foot is bigger than the other, buy shoes to fit your larger foot.
- If you have reduced sensation in your feet, take the shoes home and wear them for 30 minutes. Then remove them and examine your feet. Red areas indicate pressure and a poor fit. If you see any red areas, return the shoes. If no problems occur, gradually increase the time you wear them by one-half to one hour each day.

Don't smoke

If you have diabetes and you smoke, you're at least twice as likely as nonsmokers with diabetes to die of cardiovascular disease, such as heart disease or stroke. And you're more likely to develop circulation problems in your feet. Consider these risks:

- Smoking narrows and hardens your arteries: This increases your risk of heart attack and stroke and reduces blood flow to your legs, making it more difficult for wounds to heal.
- Smoking increases your risk of nerve damage and kidney disease.
- Smoking appears to impair your immune system, producing more colds and respiratory infections.

If you're among the approximately one in four Americans with diabetes who smoke, talk to your doctor about methods to quit smoking. And don't be discouraged if your first attempts aren't successful. Stopping smoking can take several attempts, but it's vitally important to your health.

Take a daily aspirin if your doctor approves

Studies show that taking an aspirin every day can greatly reduce the risk of heart attacks and other cardiovascular complications of people over age 40 who have type 1 or type 2 diabetes. The recommended dose is the lowest dose available. In the United States, that's 81 milligrams (mg) a day — the amount found in a baby aspirin.

When you have diabetes, you produce more "sticky" platelets that attach themselves to the inside walls of your arteries, clogging your arteries and causing blood clots to form. Clogged arteries and blood clots can lead to a heart attack or a stroke. Aspirin is an anti-clotting, anti-platelet drug that decreases the stickiness of your platelets, reducing your risk of narrowed arteries or blood clots.

It's best to take aspirin with food. A serious side effect of regular aspirin usage is that it can cause stomach irritation, bleeding or an ulcer. Enteric-coated aspirin is designed to be less erosive to the stomach in the hopes of minimizing these side effects. Once you start taking aspirin, you may notice that you bruise more easily and the bruises last longer. That's because aspirin reduces the ability of your blood platelets to seal up and heal wounds. Consult your doctor to determine the best option for your situation.

Aspirin isn't for everyone

Aspirin therapy, however, isn't for everyone. Aspirin isn't recommended for anyone under the age of 21 years because it can produce a dangerous condition called Reye's syndrome. You also shouldn't take aspirin if:

- You've had an allergic reaction to aspirin in the past
- You have a stomach ulcer
- You have liver disease
- You're taking some other drug that reduces clotting, such as warfarin (Coumadin), unless you check with your doctor

If you can't take aspirin and your doctor considers you at high risk of a heart attack or stroke, he or she may recommend a prescription blood-thinning medication.

Monitor your blood pressure

People with diabetes are about twice as likely to develop high blood pressure as individuals who don't have diabetes. Having both diabetes and high blood pressure is serious. Similar to diabetes, high blood pressure can damage your blood vessels. When you have both of these conditions and they're not under control, you increase your risk of a heart attack, stroke or other life-threatening complications.

Blood pressure is a measure of the force of circulating blood against the walls of your arteries. The higher your blood pressure, the harder your heart has to work to pump blood to all parts of your body. Blood pressure is measured as two numbers, such as 120/70 millimeters of mercury (mm Hg). The first number (upper number) is the systolic pressure, your peak pressure at the moment your heart contracts and pumps blood. The second number (lower number) is the diastolic pressure, the level of pressure when your heart relaxes to allow blood to flow into your heart.

Blood pressure goals and treatment

Adults with diabetes should keep their blood pressure below 130/80 mm Hg. If you have kidney disease, your doctor may recommend a lower blood pressure.

The same healthy habits that can improve your blood glucose — a balanced diet and regular exercise — can help reduce your blood pressure. Limiting consumption of sodium also is important. If you can't control your blood pressure with diet and exercise alone, your doctor may prescribe blood pressure lowering medication.

The ADA recommends drug therapy if your systolic pressure is at or over 140 mm Hg or your diastolic pressure is at or over 90 mm Hg. If your systolic blood pressure is 130 to 139 mm Hg or your diastolic blood pressure is 80 to 89 mm Hg, your doctor may encourage you to try making lifestyle changes over three months before prescribing drug therapy.

Drugs most often prescribed for people with diabetes include angiotensin-converting enzyme (ACE) inhibitors, angiotensin II receptor blockers and thiazide diuretics. These medications have a low rate of side effects, and they help protect your kidneys and heart, which are at high risk of damage from both diseases. Usually people with diabetes require more than two blood pressure medications to achieve their recommended goals.

Have your blood pressure checked at every doctor visit. If you have high blood pressure — especially if it's not well controlled — you may also want to monitor your blood pressure regularly at home.

Watch your cholesterol

High levels of cholesterol and triglycerides increase your risk of heart attack and stroke. So a healthy lifestyle is critically important: Focus on reducing your intake of saturated fats, trans fats and cholesterol, achieving a healthy weight, and getting regular exercise and physical activity.

Know your ABCs

If you have diabetes, work closely with your health care team to manage your ABCs and lower your risk of heart disease and stroke.

A = A1C. This test measures your average blood glucose level over the past three months. Aim for less than 7 percent. (See "A1C test," page 156.)

B = Blood pressure. Aim for less than 130/80 mm Hg.

C = Cholesterol. Aim for:
  • "Bad" (LDL) cholesterol under 100 mg/dL*
  • "Good" (HDL) cholesterol above 40 mg/dL if you're a man or above 50 mg/dL if you're a woman
  • Triglycerides under 150 mg/dL

Help manage your ABCs by making wise lifestyle choices.

*If you have cardiovascular disease, your goal for LDL cholesterol may be less than 70 mg/dL (milligrams of cholesterol per deciliter of blood).

Based on "Make the Link! Diabetes, Heart Disease and Stroke," American Diabetes Association and American College of Cardiology, 2005

If you have diabetes and you don't achieve your goals for cholesterol (see box on page 176), your doctor may prescribe a cholesterol-lowering drug called a statin, especially if:

- You're over age 40
- You're under age 40 and you have another risk factor for cardiovascular disease
- You have cardiovascular disease

Recent studies, including the Heart Protection Study, suggest that taking statins can lower the risk of heart attack or stroke in people with diabetes even if they have normal cholesterol levels. However, statin therapy isn't prescribed for women who are pregnant.

Manage stress

When you're under a lot of stress, it becomes more difficult to take good care of yourself and your diabetes. You might not eat well. You may not exercise. And you may not take your medication as prescribed. Excessive or prolonged stress also can increase production of hormones that block the effect of insulin, causing your blood glucose to rise.

Stop and think about what causes you stress. Then ask yourself if you can do anything to change the situation. If a hectic day of running from one event to another causes stress, reduce your daily commitments. If certain friends or family members cause you stress, limit the time you spend with them. If your job is stressful, look for ways to lighten the load, such as handing over some of your responsibilities to others. Also ask your health care team for advice. Some basic stress-fighting techniques include:

Making healthy food choices. Eat a well-balanced diet that includes a wide variety of healthy foods — especially fruits, vegetables and whole grains — and limit portion sizes to achieve or maintain a healthy weight.

Exercising regularly. Studies show that people who regularly exercise are better able to cope with stress and are less likely to be depressed and anxious.

Getting enough sleep. A good night's sleep refreshes you so that you're ready to tackle the day's problems.

Relief through relaxation

You can't avoid all stress, but you can minimize the effects of stress by learning healthy ways to relax. Some people relax while listening to or performing music. Others surround themselves with soothing aromas (aromatherapy). Still others benefit from practices such as yoga or meditation.

To help you get started, practice relaxed breathing (see the box on the next page). Also try progressive muscle relaxation. This technique involves relaxing a series of muscles one at a time: First, raise the tension level in a group of muscles, such as a leg or an

---

Recognizing depression

Depression can occur after periods of prolonged stress. And if you're depressed, it may affect how well you take care of yourself and your diabetes. Early treatment may keep depression from becoming more severe.

Signs and symptoms of depression include:
- Persistent sadness
- Frequent irritability
- Overwhelming feelings of anxiety
- Loss of interest or pleasure in life
- Neglect of personal responsibilities or personal care
- Changes in eating habits
- Changes in sleeping patterns
- Persistent fatigue and lack of energy
- Decreased concentration, attention and memory
- Extreme mood changes
- Feeling helpless, trapped, hopeless or worthless
- Continuous negative thinking
- Physical symptoms, such as headaches or chronic pain, that don't respond to treatment
- Increased alcohol or drug use
- Thoughts of death or suicide

Talk to your doctor or other health care provider if you have any of the above signs or symptoms for a prolonged period of time. If you find yourself frequently thinking about suicide or making a suicide plan, seek immediate medical attention.

arm, by tightening the muscles and then relaxing them. Concentrate on slowly letting the tension go in each muscle. Then move on to the next muscle group.

Practice relaxed breathing

Stress typically causes rapid, shallow breathing. If you can control your breathing, the spiraling effects of acute stress will become less intense. Practice deep relaxed breathing at least twice a day and whenever you feel tense:

- Sit comfortably with your feet flat on the floor.
- Loosen tight clothing around your abdomen and waist.
- Place your hands on your lap or at your sides.
- Relax your shoulders and close your eyes if you prefer.
- With your mouth closed, slowly breathe in through your nose while counting to six, allowing your abdomen to expand. Pause for a second.
- Then slowly exhale through your mouth as you count to six and pause again.
- Complete this breathing cycle several times.

Questions and answers

I like to travel. Can I do so safely with diabetes?
There's no reason you can't travel. The key is to make sure that you're well prepared. Carry medical identification with you and bring enough diabetes supplies and medications to last the entire trip — plus a little extra in case of scheduling changes. Don't put these items in checked bags. Keep them in your carry-on bag. Major airlines allow you to put your medicine, needles and syringes in carry-on bags as long as the medication has a pharmacy label or other professionally printed label that identifies the medication or a manufacturer's name. It's best to also have your doctor's prescription with you.

When making your reservations, you can request a special diabetic meal. Also take along food such as dried fruits or crackers to treat low blood glucose or in case you don't eat on schedule. Pack two pairs of good walking shoes, in case you have problems with one pair. As much as possible, try to follow your daily walking and eating regimen.

Instead of aspirin, will another pain reliever such as Tylenol or Advil reduce my risk of a heart attack?

No. Similar to aspirin, acetaminophen (Tylenol, others) and ibuprofen (Advil, Motrin, others) help reduce pain. But they don't have aspirin's anti-clotting capabilities. And limited evidence suggests that prolonged use of ibuprofen, naproxen (Aleve, Naprosyn, others) or ketoprofen (Orudis, Oruvail) may increase cardiovascular risk. In addition, pills known as COX-2 inhibitors (Celebrex) are linked with a higher risk of heart attack and stroke.

Should I join a support group for people with diabetes?

Many people find support groups helpful. You might consider joining a support group if you don't have a knowledgeable, understanding and supportive group of family and friends to help you. But even if your family and friends are supportive, you might benefit from the encouragement and coping strategies that members of a support group can offer. However, support groups aren't for everyone. Some people find it difficult or intimidating to interact within groups.

If you'd like to learn more about support groups, talk with your doctor, diabetes educator or dietitian, or contact the American Diabetes Association. (See "Additional resources," page 219.)

Part 5

Special issues

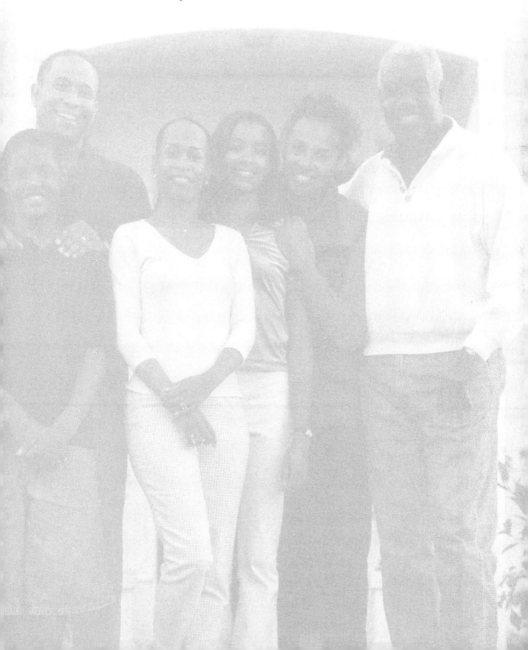

Chapter 12

Sexual health:
Issues for men and women

Sexuality is an important part of your overall well-being and another aspect of your health that's influenced by diabetes. Understanding how diabetes affects sexuality, and what you can do about it, can minimize the disease's effects and help you lead a more enjoyable life.

If you're a man, the better you control your blood glucose, the less your risk of erectile dysfunction due to nerve and blood vessel damage. If you're already experiencing erectile dysfunction, treatments are available.

If you're a woman, knowing that fluctuations in your hormone levels may affect your blood sugar (glucose) can help you better manage your diabetes during menstruation and menopause. If you're considering pregnancy, key steps before and during your pregnancy can greatly improve your chances for delivering a healthy baby, without complications.

Some people find it difficult to discuss sexual matters. But it's important to ask your doctor questions if you have concerns or problems.

Dealing with erectile dysfunction

It's estimated that more than half of men age 50 and older who have diabetes experience some degree of erectile dysfunction, sometimes called impotence. But few of them talk about it with their doctors. This is too bad because if they did, chances are good that their doctors could help them treat the condition. Erectile dysfunction refers to the inability to achieve an erection of the penis or to maintain an erection long enough for sexual intercourse.

Causes

Erectile dysfunction can result from physical or psychological factors. The most common causes in men with diabetes are physical problems due to poor blood glucose control or long-term effects of the disease. Excess blood glucose can damage the nerves and blood vessels responsible for erections, and not enough blood reaches the penis to cause an erection.

Psychological factors that can produce erectile dysfunction include stress, anxiety, fatigue or depression. They can interfere with your body's normal production of hormones and how your brain responds to them, preventing erections from occurring.

Certain medications also can cause erectile dysfunction, including some drugs used to treat high blood pressure, anxiety and depression. If you're experiencing erectile dysfunction, make sure your doctor is aware of all of the medications that you take.

When to seek medical advice

It's normal to experience erectile dysfunction on occasion. But if this problem lasts longer than two months or is recurring, see your doctor for a physical exam or for a referral to a doctor who specializes in erectile problems.

Several types of treatment are available. The cause and severity of your condition are important factors in determining the best treatment or combination of treatments for you. Don't try to combine medications or treatments on your own and don't take more than the prescribed doses. Find out if your insurance may help cover the cost of treatment.

Oral drugs

Sildenafil (Viagra), tadalafil (Cialis) and vardenafil (Levitra) are phosphodiesterase (fos-fo-di-ES-ter-ase) type 5 inhibitors, also called PDE5 inhibitors. For some men with erectile dysfunction resulting from diabetes, these medications can improve sexual function, but they aren't effective for everyone.

Unlike other treatments for erectile dysfunction, these drugs produce a more natural erection instead of an artificial one. These drugs can help you respond to sexual or psychological stimulation by relaxing the smooth muscle tissue in the penis, which in turn increases blood flow in the penis and makes it easier for you to achieve and maintain an erection. All of these medications are taken about an hour before sexual intercourse. These drugs are effective for varying lengths of time (from about four to 36 hours) and shouldn't be used more often than directed by your doctor.

Safety issues. These drugs aren't safe for all men. You shouldn't take these drugs if you're also taking nitrates, such as nitroglycerin. If these drugs are taken together with some blood pressure and prostate medications, this mix of medicine can substantially lower your blood pressure and produce a fatal heart attack.

This class of drugs can cause other side effects. They may produce facial flushing, which generally lasts no more than five to 10 minutes. You may also experience a temporary mild headache or an upset stomach. Higher doses can produce short-term visual problems: a slight bluish tinge to objects, blurred vision and increased light sensitivity. These effects generally go away a few hours after taking the drug. Specific instructions vary for each drug, so review the instructions with your doctor before taking any of these medications.

Alprostadil

There are two treatments that involve using a drug called alprostadil (al-PROS-tuh-dil). Alprostadil is a synthetic version of the chemical prostaglandin E. As with the oral drugs, this medication helps relax smooth muscle tissue in the penis, which enhances the blood flow needed for an erection. There are two ways to use alprostadil: by self-administered intraurethral (in-tra-yoo-REE-thrul) therapy or self-injection therapy.

Self-administered intraurethral therapy. This method's trade name is Medicated Urethral System for Erection (MUSE). It involves using a disposable applicator to insert a tiny suppository, about half the size of a grain of rice, into the tip of your penis. The suppository, placed about two inches into your urethra, is absorbed by erectile tissue in your penis, increasing the blood flow that causes an erection. Some men find this method uncomfortable. Side effects may include pain, minor bleeding or burning in the urethra, or dizziness.

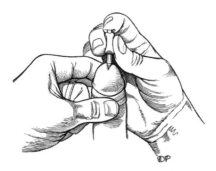

Self-administered intraurethral therapy involves inserting a tiny suppository into the tip of your penis to help relax smooth muscle tissue and increase blood flow to the penis.

Self-injection therapy. With this method, you use a fine needle to inject alprostadil (Caverject, Edex) into the base or side of your penis. This generally produces an erection in five to 20 minutes that lasts about an hour. Alprostadil is an effective treatment for many men. Pain from the injection site is usually minor. Other side effects may include bleeding from the injection, prolonged erection or, rarely, formation of fibrous tissue at the injection site. Injecting a mixture of alprostadil with either of the prescription drugs papaverine or phentolamine (Regitine) may improve effectiveness.

Self-injection therapy involves injecting medication directly into a specific area of the penis to increase blood flow and cause an erection.

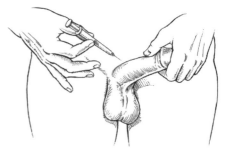

Vacuum devices

Many men turn to vacuum devices when medication is ineffective or its side effects are too bothersome. This treatment involves the use of an external vacuum and one or more rubber bands (tension rings). You begin by placing a hollow plastic tube (available by prescription) over your penis. You then use a hand pump to create a vacuum in the tube and pull blood into your penis, producing an erection. You then slip off an elastic ring (mounted on the base of the plastic tube), pulling it around the base of your penis. This traps the blood inside your penis, allowing you to keep your erection once the tube is removed. You should remove the ring within 30 minutes to restore normal blood flow to your penis. If you don't, you could damage penile tissue.

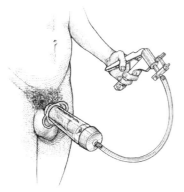

A vacuum device has a hand pump to draw blood into the penis, creating an erection. An elastic ring placed at the base of the penis keeps it erect.

Penile implants

If you've tried medication or a vacuum device and it hasn't worked or has been uncomfortable, you might consider one of the surgical implants described below. However, this type of treatment is often expensive, and as with any surgery, there is a small risk of complications, such as infection.

Semirigid, bendable rod. A semirigid, bendable rod type of implant is the easiest to use and the least likely to malfunction. Two hard but flexible rods made of wires and covered with silicone or polyurethane are placed inside your penis. They give you a permanent erection. You bend your penis down toward your body to hide the erection and bend it up to have sexual intercourse. Although it takes some getting used to, this implant requires less surgical time than other implants do, has no mechanical parts to break and has a high success rate.

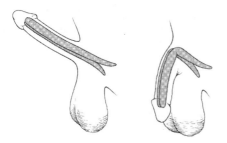

With semirigid implants, the penis is always erect. To hide the erection, the implanted rods are bent down.

Inflatable. These implants work more naturally than the semirigid rods. Instead of having a permanent erection, you produce an erection only when you want one.

One version includes two hollow cylinders that are placed into your penis. These cylinders are connected to a tiny pump in your scrotum and to a reservoir in either your scrotum or your lower abdomen. When you squeeze the pump, fluid from the reservoir fills the cylinders and produces an erection. The device is easily concealed and very effective, but it's more likely than other implants to have mechanical failure.

Another version doesn't involve a pump. Instead, a device near the head of your penis controls the flow of fluid inside the cylinders. To get an erection, you squeeze the head of your penis. This releases fluid into the cylinders. To shift the fluid back into place and produce a limp penis, you bend the implant and press a release valve.

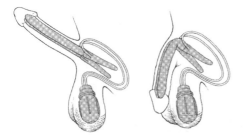

With some inflatable implants, you squeeze a pump, causing fluid from a reservoir to fill inflatable cylinders in the penis and produce an erection. When an erection isn't wanted, the fluid is directed back to the reservoir.

Counseling

Erectile dysfunction typically causes anxiety, stress, misunderstanding and frustration to both partners. Psychological factors can play a significant role in this disorder and can be effectively treated with the aid of a psychiatrist, psychologist or other licensed therapist with experience in treating sexual problems. Pursuing both the psychological and physical factors of erectile dysfunction is important to a successful treatment outcome.

Menstruation and blood glucose

Your ovaries produce the hormones estrogen and progesterone, which regulate your menstrual, or reproductive, cycle. As the hormone levels fluctuate during the cycle, so can your blood glucose.

Most women who have menstruation-related changes in blood glucose notice it in the seven to 14 days before bleeding begins. Blood glucose generally stabilizes a day or two after the period starts. These changes tend to be more noticeable in women with premenstrual syndrome (PMS).

Premenstrual syndrome is a condition that occurs in some women about a week before menstruation. Symptoms include mood swings, tender breasts, bloating, lethargy, food cravings and lack of concentration. Giving in to cravings for carbohydrates and fats also can make blood glucose control more difficult.

High blood glucose can also lead to other problems, such as:
- Yeast infections of the vagina
- Irregular menstrual periods
- Loss of skin sensation around the vaginal area

What you can do

Keep a log: Record your blood glucose levels on a daily basis. Also record the day your period begins and the day it ends. Look for patterns in your blood glucose levels, especially the week before your period. Then talk with your doctor. Your doctor may recommend changes in your medication dose or schedule, or your eating or exercise regimens, to make up for swings in your blood glucose.

Menopause and diabetes: Unique challenges

Menopause — and the years leading up to it when your body gradually produces less estrogen and progesterone (perimenopause) — may present unique challenges if you have diabetes. When 12 months have passed since your last period, you've reached menopause. Menopause most often occurs between the ages of 45 and 55, but it can occur at younger or older ages.

As you approach menopause, your ovaries gradually stop producing estrogen and progesterone. How these hormonal changes affect blood glucose may vary, depending on the individual. However, many women notice that their blood glucose levels are more variable (increases and decreases) and less predictable than before. These hormonal changes as well as swings in your blood glucose levels can contribute to menopausal symptoms such as mood changes, fatigue and hot flashes.

Similar symptoms

You may mistake menopausal symptoms such as hot flashes, moodiness and short-term memory loss for symptoms of low blood glucose. If you incorrectly assume these symptoms are due to low blood glucose, you may consume unnecessary calories to try to raise your blood glucose and cause it to go too high.

Because of your diabetes, however, you may have stronger and more frequent episodes of low blood glucose, especially at night. This can make sleeping even more difficult if it's already interrupted by hot flashes and night sweats from menopause.

The combination of menopause and diabetes can also cause other problems, such as:

- **Vaginal dryness.** Decreased blood flow to the vagina causes its lining to become thin and dry.
- **Yeast infections.** Increased levels of glucose in vaginal mucus and vaginal secretions that are less acidic and protective increase susceptibility to such infections.
- **Urinary tract infections.** Thinning of the lining of the bladder increases susceptibility to infections.

Although it's easy to confuse the symptoms of menopause and diabetes, and to treat your diabetes inappropriately as a result, you can take steps to reduce such problems.

What you can do

To help manage your diabetes during menopause:

Measure your blood glucose frequently. You may have to check your blood glucose level three or four times a day, and occasionally during the night. If you keep a log of your levels and symptoms, it can help your doctor make necessary adjustments in your treatment.

Work with your doctor to adjust diabetes medications. If your blood glucose increases, you may need to increase the dosage of your diabetes medications or begin taking a new medication. This is especially likely if you gain weight or reduce your level of physical activity. If your blood glucose decreases, you may need to reduce your dosages. Your need for insulin, for example, may significantly decline. If you gain weight or stop exercising, however, your dosages may remain the same, because additional weight and lack of physical activity increase resistance to insulin.

Ask your doctor if you need a cholesterol-lowering drug. If you have diabetes, you're at increased risk of heart and blood vessel (cardiovascular) disease. High levels of total and LDL ("bad") cholesterol add to this risk, as does menopause. As a result, many people with diabetes need a cholesterol-lowering drug — usually a statin — to reduce their risk of heart attack, stroke and other cardiovascular diseases. (See "Know your ABCs," page 176, for target cholesterol levels.)

Get help for menopausal symptoms. You may want to see a gynecologist for help with especially intense hot flashes or vaginal dryness and thinning. If you're having problems with vaginal symptoms, for example, your doctor can prescribe treatments to help restore moisture. And antibiotics can help treat urinary tract infections. If weight gain is a problem, consider consulting with a dietitian to help review your meal plans.

Is it safe to take hormone therapy?

For some women, hormone therapy (HT) helps ease troublesome symptoms of menopause, such as hot flashes and night sweats. Women may take a form of HT that provides both estrogen and progestin (such as Prempro) or a form that provides estrogen alone (such as Premarin), for women who no longer have a uterus.

Contrary to what doctors thought years ago, recent large controlled studies based on the Women's Health Initiative show that hormone therapy does *not* reduce the risk of heart disease in postmenopausal women. These studies show that the combination form (estrogen plus progestin) of HT can actually increase the risk of a heart attack and breast cancer, and confirmed that both forms of HT increase the risk of stroke. And if you have diabetes or prediabetes, you're already at a higher risk of heart attack and stroke.

For many women in the studies, combination HT didn't provide a meaningful improvement in quality-of-life measures such as sleep, emotional health, general health, physical functioning and sexual satisfaction. Despite these studies, unanswered questions remain about the safety, risks and benefits of hormone therapy.

Whether to take hormone therapy is an individual, complex decision, based on your health history and health risks. Talk with your doctor about the benefits and risks of hormone therapy and possible alternatives if you're dealing with hot flashes and other symptoms of menopause.

Diabetes and pregnancy

You have diabetes and are thinking about becoming pregnant. You look forward to becoming a mother and want to give birth to a healthy baby. Ready for some good news? Women with diabetes who control their blood glucose before they're pregnant and during their pregnancy have almost the same chance of having a healthy baby as do women without diabetes. Your blood glucose level should be in good control for three to six months before you try to get pregnant.

Why it's best to plan your pregnancy

To prevent diabetes-related complications for both you and your baby, make sure your blood glucose is under control before you become pregnant. Your blood glucose not only affects your health, it affects your baby's health, too.

Your baby's organs form during the first six to eight weeks of pregnancy. But you probably won't know you're pregnant until your baby has been growing for two to four weeks. So if you don't plan your pregnancy and you have poor blood glucose control, your baby's risk of birth defects is much higher. Birth defects can affect your baby's brain, heart and kidneys.

To help prevent birth defects, your doctor will recommend that you take a multivitamin with folic acid each day, ideally starting three months before you get pregnant, and a prenatal vitamin throughout your pregnancy.

Planning before pregnancy

Your doctor and your health care team can help you achieve good blood glucose control and prepare your body for a healthy pregnancy. But it's up to you to follow through with the plan. Here's what your plan before pregnancy may include.

Birth control. Practicing birth control before pregnancy allows you and your health care team to choose the safest time to have a baby.

Complete physical exam. A physical exam helps identify health conditions that may increase your risk of complications. These conditions include high blood pressure and eye, nerve or kidney disease. Because pregnancy may aggravate these conditions, your doctor will want to treat them before you become pregnant.

Control over your blood glucose. Good blood glucose control is essential if you're planning to get pregnant, so that you can reduce your risk of diabetes-related complications for you and your baby.

If you have type 1 diabetes, you may require intensive insulin therapy to keep your glucose within a normal or near-normal range (tight control). This includes frequent monitoring of your blood glucose, a combination of different types of insulin, and adjusting your doses based on your blood glucose levels, diet and changes in your routine. If you have type 2 diabetes, you may have to switch to intensive insulin therapy to get better control of your blood glucose. (See "Intensive insulin therapy," page 107.)

Your doctor will tell you the target range for your blood glucose as you prepare for pregnancy. When your A1C test result reaches near-normal levels, under 7 percent, your doctor may recommend that you stop using birth control. (See "A1C test," page 156.)

Meal planning. A healthy meal plan helps you maintain normal or near-normal blood glucose levels. You may need to work with a dietitian to modify your meal plan if you're having trouble keeping your blood glucose within your target range or if you need to manage your weight. Artificial sweeteners may be a concern. The effects on the fetus are unknown, so it's best during your pregnancy to avoid products containing saccharin and aspartame.

Regular exercise. Regular exercise improves blood glucose control and weight management. But start slowly and progress gradually if you haven't been exercising. If you take insulin, don't forget to test your blood glucose before and after you exercise to avoid low blood glucose.

When you become pregnant

Like most women, you're probably experiencing the joys and fears of having a baby. But you're concerned about the effects diabetes can have on your body, on labor and on delivery, and you're concerned about the health of your baby.

Because of your diabetes, you'll have extra challenges to deal with during your pregnancy. But the most important challenge is keeping your blood glucose under tight control. With the help of your health care team, you can monitor your blood glucose and avoid complications as your pregnancy progresses. In addition to the health care team members listed on page 154, your team may include:

- An obstetrician who has special training in handling high-risk pregnancies and pregnancies of women with diabetes
- A pediatrician or neonatologist with expertise in treating babies born to women with diabetes (a pediatrician specializes in the treatment of children, and a neonatologist is a pediatrician who specializes in the care of sick babies)

If you live in a small town or a rural area and don't have easy access to specialists, ask your doctor about his or her experience treating pregnant women with diabetes. Find out if this doctor has access to a specialist at a nearby university or metropolitan area. Your doctor may have you visit a specialist once during your pregnancy and consult with the specialist during your pregnancy.

Tight control. As in the pre-pregnancy stage, during your pregnancy your chief goal is to keep your blood glucose under tight control. Your doctor will tell you what your target blood glucose range is.

If you have type 2 diabetes, you'll probably stop taking oral medications and take insulin to manage your blood glucose while you're pregnant. One reason is that intensive insulin therapy can achieve tighter control of your blood glucose. Another is that the safety

Tight glucose control reduces birth defects

Blood glucose control is crucial not only to your health but to the health of your unborn child. If during the first six to eight weeks of your baby's development — when your baby's heart, lungs, kidneys and brain are being formed — your blood glucose is too high, your baby is at increased risk of birth defects. A high level of ketones in your blood (diabetic ketoacidosis) also can cause miscarriage.

Later in pregnancy, uncontrolled blood glucose can lead to premature birth or stillbirth or other problems. Fortunately, most of these problems are preventable or treatable. (See "Complications from uncontrolled blood glucose," page 200.)

of oral diabetes medications for pregnant women and unborn babies is unknown when taken during all nine months of pregnancy.

If you need to switch to insulin therapy, your health care team will teach you how to take insulin. The team will also tell you how often to check your blood glucose.

What to expect during your pregnancy

Here's what can happen as your pregnancy progresses.

First trimester. During the first 10 to 12 weeks of your pregnancy, you'll probably see your obstetrician every one to two weeks. This is the time that your baby's organs are developing, so your blood glucose needs to be as close to normal as possible to prevent birth defects. Frequent blood glucose monitoring can help you do this. Because your need for insulin may drop slightly during this time, be alert to signs of low blood glucose. If morning sickness makes you miserable, talk with your doctor about medication to treat nausea.

Second trimester. The second trimester is when you'll likely receive an ultrasound to check the health of your baby. Your doctor will also keep track of your weight gain. If your weight is normal when you start your pregnancy, research suggests a total gain of 25 to 35 pounds is healthiest for you and your baby. If you're too thin, you may need to gain more. If you're obese, you may need to work with a dietitian to limit your weight gain.

If you take insulin, expect your insulin requirements to rise gradually to about week 20 and then accelerate dramatically. Hormones made by the placenta to help your baby grow block the effect of your insulin, so you'll need significantly more to compensate. At this stage of your pregnancy, it's also important to see an eye specialist. Damage to the small blood vessels in your eyes can progress during pregnancy.

Third trimester. During the final three months of your pregnancy, you'll need careful monitoring. The doctor will check for complications that can occur during the late stage of any pregnancy, such as high blood pressure, swollen ankles from fluid buildup and kidney problems. Your doctor may also recommend that you have your eyes examined again to check for eye damage.

Because women with diabetes are more likely to give birth to babies who weigh more than 9 pounds, you may receive another ultrasound to assess the size and health of your baby. At this stage, any potential problem for you or your baby may prompt early delivery.

Labor and delivery
Your health care team will help you determine the best time and safest method to deliver your baby. Delivering your baby at home with a nurse midwife generally isn't recommended because of the increased potential for problems due to your diabetes.

As long as your blood glucose remains normal, and you and your baby don't experience complications, you can expect a normal vaginal delivery. During labor, your blood glucose will be closely monitored to prevent a large decrease or increase in your glucose levels. Because your body is working so hard and using glucose as energy, you'll likely need less insulin.

What to watch out for

During your pregnancy, you'll need to be alert for hypoglycemia, hyperglycemia and ketone buildup. For signs and symptoms of these conditions, see Chapter 2.

Low blood glucose (hypoglycemia). Tight blood glucose control can improve your chances of having a healthy pregnancy, but it also puts you at risk of low blood glucose. If episodes of hypoglycemia are frequent and severe, your health and that of your baby is at risk.

High blood glucose (hyperglycemia). High blood glucose can occur if your body doesn't have enough insulin, you overeat or you exercise less than you planned. Stress or illness, such as a cold or influenza, also can cause high blood glucose.

Ketone buildup (diabetic ketoacidosis). Diabetic ketoacidosis is caused by increased levels of ketones, blood acids that your body produces when your cells lack insulin and can't use glucose. Ketones can build up in your blood and endanger your health and that of your baby.

If there are complications or your baby is too large for a safe vaginal delivery, your baby may be delivered by Caesarean section through an incision in your lower abdominal and uterine walls. Regardless of the delivery method, the result for most women who've maintained good blood glucose control is a healthy baby.

Following delivery, your insulin needs will decrease. However, it may take weeks to months before your body changes are complete and you return to your normal medication regimen.

Gestational diabetes

Gestational diabetes only occurs during the time you're pregnant, generally in the second or third trimester. Like other forms of diabetes, gestational diabetes causes your blood glucose to become too high. If untreated or uncontrolled, gestational diabetes can result in health problems for you and your baby.

During pregnancy, your placenta — the organ that supplies your baby with nutrients through the umbilical cord — produces hormones that prevent insulin from doing its job. These hormones are vital to preserving your pregnancy. Yet they also make your cells more resistant to insulin.

Pregnancy and different types of diabetes

It's important to make the distinction between type 1, type 2 and gestational (jes-TAY-shun-ul) diabetes, although all three types require close monitoring and tight glucose control during pregnancy. Type 1 or type 2 diabetes develops before or after pregnancy. Gestational diabetes occurs only during pregnancy.

Gestational diabetes is caused by an increased production of the hormones estrogen and progesterone during pregnancy. This type of diabetes also differs in that it disappears immediately following delivery. However, gestational diabetes increases your risk of developing type 2 diabetes later in life.

Rarely, some women develop type 1 or type 2 diabetes during pregnancy. In most cases, the condition is initially diagnosed as gestational diabetes. But unlike gestational diabetes, blood glucose levels don't improve after the pregancy. Glucose levels remain high, requiring daily insulin.

As your placenta grows larger in the second and third trimesters, it secretes even more of these hormones, further increasing insulin resistance. Normally, your pancreas responds by producing enough extra insulin to overcome this resistance. But you may need up to three times as much insulin as normal, and sometimes your pancreas simply can't keep up. When this happens, too little glucose gets into your cells and too much stays in your blood.

Gestational diabetes usually occurs about the 20th to 24th week of pregnancy and can be measured by the 24th to 28th week of pregnancy. After your baby is born and placental hormones disappear from your bloodstream, your blood glucose levels should quickly return to normal.

Most women don't experience any signs or symptoms of gestational diabetes. When they do occur, signs and symptoms may include excessive thirst and increased urination.

Risk factors. Any woman can develop gestational diabetes, but factors that increase your risk include:

- Age over 25
- Family history of gestational diabetes
- Gestational diabetes in a previous pregnancy
- Being overweight before pregnancy
- Black American, Hispanic or American Indian race (for reasons that aren't clear)
- Unexplained stillbirth
- Delivering a baby more than 9 pounds

Screening and diagnosis. In some places, screening for gestational diabetes is a routine part of prenatal care. To screen for gestational diabetes, most doctors recommend a glucose challenge test. This test is usually done between 24 and 28 weeks of pregnancy, because the condition usually can't be detected until then. However, if your doctor thinks you're at high risk, the test may be done earlier. The glucose challenge test is a modified version of the oral glucose tolerance test, explained on page 17.

Treatment. Controlling your blood glucose is essential to keeping your baby healthy and avoiding complications. Monitoring your blood glucose is a key part of your treatment program to see if your blood glucose is staying within a normal range. Most women with

Complications from uncontrolled blood glucose

Most women with diabetes (any type) deliver healthy babies. However, untreated or uncontrolled blood glucose levels can cause serious problems.

Complications that may affect your baby

Keeping your blood glucose levels within a normal range can reduce the risk of complications, such as:

Macrosomia. Extra glucose can cross the placenta and end up in your baby's blood. When that happens, your baby's pancreas makes extra insulin to process the extra glucose, and this can cause your baby to grow too large (macrosomia).

Shoulder dystocia. If you have a very large baby, the shoulders may be too big to move through the birth canal, a potentially life-threatening emergency known as shoulder dystocia (dis-TOE-shuh). In most cases, doctors can perform maneuvers to free the baby.

Hypoglycemia. Sometimes, babies of mothers with diabetes develop low blood glucose (hypoglycemia) shortly after birth. That's because they've been receiving large amounts of blood glucose from their mothers, and their own insulin production is high. Hypoglycemia is easily detected and treated.

gestational diabetes are able to control their blood glucose with diet and exercise, but some may also need insulin.

Results of a recent study support more aggressive treatment in women with gestational diabetes. Researchers compared pregnancy outcomes in two groups. One group received aggressive treatment to maintain tight glucose control — dietary advice, more frequent blood glucose monitoring and insulin injections for glucose levels above a desired range.

The other group received routine care, glucose wasn't monitored as often, and they may or may not have used insulin. The women who received aggressive treatment with insulin maintained tighter glucose control and developed significantly fewer childbirth problems than did the women under routine care. These results will likely affect future medical management of gestational diabetes.

Respiratory distress syndrome. Babies born prematurely to mothers with diabetes are more likely to develop respiratory distress syndrome, a condition that makes breathing difficult.

Jaundice. Jaundice is a yellowish discoloration of the skin and the whites of the eyes from a buildup of old blood cells that aren't being cleared away fast enough by your baby's liver. This is easily treated, but requires careful monitoring.

Stillbirth or death. If the mother's diabetes goes undetected, a baby has an increased risk of stillbirth or death as a newborn.

Complications that may affect you

If you have diabetes, you may be at risk of:

Preeclampsia. A condition called preeclampsia (pree-ih-KLAMP-see-uh) is primarily characterized by a significant increase in blood pressure. Left untreated, it can lead to serious, even deadly complications for the mother and baby.

Having a C-section. Having diabetes isn't a reason to schedule a Caesarean delivery, commonly called a C-section, but your doctor may recommend one if your baby has macrosomia.

In addition, a recent small study indicates that glyburide, an oral drug, may be safe for women with gestational diabetes after the first trimester. There was no increase in complications. But glyburide is not FDA-approved for the treatment of diabetes during pregnancy. More studies in larger groups are needed to confirm this finding.

After delivery. To make sure that your glucose level has returned to normal after your baby is born, you'll typically have your blood glucose checked often after delivery and again in six weeks. Once you've had gestational diabetes, continue to have your blood glucose tested at least once a year. And remember: The very steps you're taking to control your blood glucose — such as eating a healthy diet and getting regular exercise — may also help prevent you from developing type 2 diabetes in the future.

Questions and answers

I have type 1 diabetes, which was diagnosed during pregnancy. What are the chances that my child will develop it, too?
A genetic counselor can help you predict the chances that your child will develop type 1 diabetes, but the risk is slightly higher than if you didn't have diabetes. (See "How does family history affect your risk of diabetes?" page 20.)

Why does my blood glucose level drop after sexual intercourse?
Your body responds to sexual intercourse as it does to exercise. Just as blood glucose drops during and following exercise due to increased need for energy (glucose) by your muscles and tissues, so it does with sexual intercourse. Testing your blood glucose before having sexual intercourse can save you an episode of low blood glucose afterward. To prevent a decrease in blood glucose, you might eat something before or immediately after you have intercourse.

How do I know if my erectile dysfunction is due to physical or psychological factors?
A sudden inability to maintain an erection is usually related to psychological factors, such as stress, or medications, such as anti-depressants. In addition, if you still experience erections while you sleep, your erectile dysfunction is probably due to psychological factors. A gradual loss of erection, on the other hand, is more likely to be related to physical factors, such as nerve and blood vessel disease. If the cause of your erectile dysfunction is uncertain, various tests can help identify its source. Discuss your concerns with your doctor to find out your treatment options.

Chapter 13

If your child has diabetes

If your son or daughter was recently diagnosed with diabetes, chances are you've launched a frenzied mission to find out everything you can about managing this condition. If that's the case, take a step back and remind yourself that the last thing your child needs now is an exhausted, stressed-out parent.

It's important to learn as much as you can about diabetes and its management. As you gain knowledge, you'll also gain confidence that your child can still thrive with diabetes. But it takes time to get a grasp on diabetes and to develop the best treatment plan for your child. Your starting point will depend on whether your child has type 1 or type 2 diabetes.

Type 1 diabetes

More than 13,000 children are diagnosed with type 1 diabetes each year in the United States. As noted in Chapter 1, in type 1 diabetes, the pancreas produces little if any insulin. Without this hormone available to move blood sugar (glucose) into the body's muscles and tissue, excess glucose accumulates in the bloodstream. Untreated, diabetes can cause serious organ damage and even death.

Signs and symptoms of type 1 diabetes

Signs and symptoms of type 1 diabetes usually develop quickly, over a period of weeks, in children and teenagers. The first indication in babies and young children may be a yeast infection that causes a severe diaper rash. Fatigue or irritability is common and should raise your suspicion when associated with the most common warning signs of:

- Frequent urination
- Intense thirst
- Constant hunger
- Unexplained weight loss

Testing for type 1 diabetes

If type 1 diabetes is suspected, your child's doctor will probably obtain a random blood glucose test at the initial visit to check for an abnormally high level of glucose. Random means any time of day, without the need for fasting. A result of 200 milligrams per deciliter (mg/dL) or greater will confirm the diagnosis.

In some circumstances, the doctor may recommend a fasting blood glucose test. Before having blood drawn for this test, your child will be instructed not to eat or drink for at least eight hours — typically, overnight. After a fast, a blood glucose level under 100 mg/dL is considered normal. A glucose level from 100 to 125 mg/dL is called prediabetes, which indicates a high risk of developing diabetes. If it's 126 mg/dL or higher on two separate tests, the doctor will diagnose diabetes. If your child is diagnosed with type 1 diabetes, it's best to have an evaluation by an experienced diabetes team, including a pediatric endocrinologist (a doctor who specializes in treating children who have diabetes).

The doctor may order additional tests to check for a high ketone level in your child's urine or blood. Ketones are toxic acids that the body produces when it's not getting enough glucose and resorts to breaking down stored fat. Excess ketones can cause a life-threatening condition called diabetic ketoacidosis (kee-toe-ass-ih-DOE-sis), or DKA. With prompt treatment this condition can be reversed. Children with DKA initially need treatment in a hospital. However, some children with mild DKA may be quickly and effectively treated with insulin therapy without the need for hospitalization. (See "High level of ketones," page 25.)

Treatments for type 1 diabetes

All people with type 1 diabetes depend on insulin therapy to live. Your child may take insulin with a syringe, an insulin pen or an insulin pump. (See Chapter 7, "Insulin therapy.")

Goals for glucose control in children and teens with type 1 diabetes

Typical glucose control targets for different age groups are listed below. But the goals for your child may differ, based on individual needs, especially if your child has problems with low blood glucose (hypoglycemia).

You or your child can use a blood glucose meter to see if mealtime and bedtime glucose levels are on track. At least every three months, the doctor will likely give your child an A1C test, which is a blood test. The result indicates your child's average blood glucose level over the past two to three months.

Age range	Blood glucose goal before meals	Blood glucose goal at bedtime and overnight	A1C goal
Toddlers and preschoolers 5 years and younger	100 to 180 mg/dL*	110 to 200 mg/dL	No lower than 7.5 percent and no higher than 8.5 percent
Children 6 through 12 years	90 to 180 mg/dL	100 to 180 mg/dL	Less than 8 percent
Teenagers 13 through 19 years	90 to 130 mg/dL	90 to 150 mg/dL	Less than 7.5 percent**

*Milligrams of glucose per deciliter of blood
**Or less than 7 percent if this lower goal doesn't result in excessive hypoglycemia
Source: American Diabetes Association, 2005

The goal of insulin therapy is to bring blood glucose levels as near to normal as possible. Target blood glucose ranges for children and adolescents taking insulin may differ from the ranges set for adults. Tight blood glucose control increases the risk of low blood glucose (hypoglycemia), and frequent instances of hypoglycemia can harm a young child's developing brain. Near-normal blood glucose levels may be hard to achieve in children and teens. Your doctor will choose a blood glucose target range according to your child's medical needs and individual situation.

The initial insulin dosage is based on weight, age, activity level and whether puberty has started. Your doctor can regularly assist in adjusting your child's insulin program as these factors change. However, self-management skills are critically important for optimal control of diabetes, and both you and — when old enough — your child need to learn how to adjust insulin doses. With the help of your doctor and diabetes educator, you and your child can become comfortable making adjustments in insulin doses to manage the expected changes in insulin needs as your child grows.

In children and teens, the insulin regimens most often used are:

Multiple daily injections (MDIs). This regimen consists of a rapid- or short-acting insulin taken before meals and snacks as well as a long-acting insulin taken once a day to provide a baseline amount throughout the day.

Split-mixed program. This is a mixture of rapid- or short-acting insulin and intermediate-acting insulin in one injection, usually given twice each day.

An insulin pump. A programmable pump worn outside the body provides a continuous infusion of rapid- or short-acting insulin. Studies show that insulin pumps are as safe and effective as injections, even for many infants and toddlers. Ask your child's doctor how well the pump has worked for other children the same age as your child. Before deciding to use a pump, call your insurance provider. Pumps are more expensive than injections, but many plans cover much of the cost.

Type 2 diabetes

Type 2 diabetes used to be considered an adult disease. It was even referred to as adult-onset diabetes. No more. Today, a significant number of type 2 cases are diagnosed in children.

Why? Obesity plays a major role. Over the past three decades, the rate of childhood obesity has more than doubled for children and teenagers. Those extra pounds carry an increased risk of type 2 diabetes. Today, most children and teenagers diagnosed with type 2 diabetes are overweight. Additional risk factors include:

- Family history: Risk increases if a parent or sibling or other close relative has type 2 diabetes, but it's difficult to tell if this is learned behavior or genetics or both.
- Race: Black Americans, Hispanic Americans, American Indians, Asian Americans and Pacific Islanders are at higher risk for unclear reasons.
- Signs of insulin resistance: These are signs such as high blood pressure, polycystic ovarian syndrome or abnormal levels of blood fats (lipids).

Signs and symptoms of type 2 diabetes

Unlike type 1 diabetes, in which the symptoms typically develop quickly, the signs and symptoms of type 2 diabetes often appear gradually. These may include:

- Frequent urination
- Intense thirst
- Constant hunger
- Unexplained weight loss
- Fatigue
- Blurred vision
- Frequent infections
- Slow-healing sores

Most children with type 2 diabetes have patches of dark, velvety skin in the folds and creases of their bodies, usually in the armpits and neck. This condition, called acanthosis nigricans (ak-an-THO-sis NI-grih-kuns), is a sign of insulin resistance and increases the probability that your child has type 2 diabetes.

However, some children with type 2 diabetes don't have any symptoms. To diagnose the disease before it does serious damage, experts recommend testing all children and adolescents who are at high risk, even if they're symptom-free. One key risk factor is having a body mass index (BMI) greater than the 85th percentile for your child's age and sex. The BMI is a measurement based on a formula that takes into account weight and height to determine if your child has an unhealthy percentage of body fat.

If your child is overweight and has two of the risk factors previously noted — overweight, family history, high-risk race or signs of insulin resistance — ask your doctor about scheduling a diabetes screening.

Doctors usually use a fasting blood glucose test to diagnose type 2 diabetes. Your child will need to avoid food and liquid for at least eight hours before having blood drawn. If the test measures a blood glucose level of 126 mg/dL or higher on two separate tests, your child has diabetes.

Prediabetes

If a fasting blood glucose test indicates a level from 100 to 125 mg/dL, your child may be diagnosed with prediabetes. Many people with prediabetes eventually develop type 2 diabetes.

Studies have shown that adults with prediabetes who make dramatic improvements to their lifestyle, including eating healthier foods and exercising more, may prevent type 2 diabetes from developing. Children and teens with prediabetes can reduce their risk by making these same changes. Ask your child's doctor for guidance. In addition, ask how often your child should be screened for diabetes.

Whether your child has prediabetes or diabetes, developing healthy eating habits, increasing physical activity and getting regular exercise are vital to prevention and disease management.

Treatments for type 2 diabetes

Some children and teenagers with type 2 diabetes can manage their blood glucose with diet and exercise alone, but many need medical treatment. In the United States, most children with type 2 diabetes are treated with insulin, although many are treated with oral drugs that lower blood glucose. The decision about which treatment is best depends on the child, the level of blood glucose and whether there are other health problems.

Metformin, explained in Chapter 8, is the only oral medication that's approved for children and adolescents (age 10 and older) with type 2 diabetes. It's an effective option for many people with diabetes, but some brands are only for use in adults. In addition, metformin isn't safe for anyone with liver, kidney or heart failure, and it may cause gastrointestinal problems.

Caring for medical needs

Leaving your child in the care of someone else can be nerve-racking for any parent. If your child has diabetes, you might be even more fearful. But both you and your child are likely to feel more secure knowing that people outside the family can be relied on to help manage diabetes. And your child will build self-confidence from handling diabetes care when you're not around. So take a deep breath, and then take action.

Creating a diabetes care plan

Sit down with your diabetes educator to create a care plan that maps out your child's treatment regimen and how to respond to high or low blood glucose. Then, meet with school or child care personnel to go over the plan in detail. Note the names of adults who will be primarily responsible for helping your child check blood glucose and take medications. This usually involves the school nurse.

Ask the school nurse or an administrator to help you share the plan with all adults who'll be supervising your child during the day, including teachers, office staff, coaches and bus drivers. Your child's diabetes educator or doctor may be able to help you train school and child care staff to perform diabetes care tasks.

Blood glucose monitoring

Regular blood glucose tests are the only way to know with confidence whether your child's treatment program is working. Whether they have type 1 or type 2 diabetes, children and teenagers who use insulin may need four or more blood glucose checks each day. Your child's doctor can help you determine the best testing schedule.

Each time you perform a blood glucose test, log the results in a record book. (See "Recording your results," page 48.) Keep a separate record book at your child's school for tracking results during the day. Young children will need an adult's help to maintain school record books, but children age 8 and older may be able to log results on their own.

The information you record will help you see how food, physical activity, illness and other factors affect your child's blood glucose. You'll soon start to see patterns that will help your doctor develop the best treatment program for your child.

Young children in particular may have a hard time recognizing the signs and symptoms of low blood glucose (hypoglycemia), explained in Chapter 2. Teach your child — and any caregivers — that if there's any doubt, check the blood glucose.

Regardless of age, getting used to frequent glucose checks can be challenging for your child — and for you. Focus on reassuring (rather than scolding) your child when he or she resists testing because it's uncomfortable. Allow your young child some decisions, even if it's as simple as choosing the spot for the glucose check. Consider simple rewards, such as stickers (not food). Ask your health care team how to approach this task, including how to deal with the emotional challenges you may face.

Involving your child in diabetes care

Encourage your child's active participation in meetings about diabetes care. Eventually, your child will need to take on total responsibility for managing diabetes. You can start working toward that goal from the beginning by asking your child to help with care tasks in age-appropriate ways.

The extent to which your child is ready to participate depends on age, abilities and willingness. Here's a general idea of what you can aim for, but ask your child's doctor for guidance because children develop at different rates:

Ages 2 to 3. Your child may be able to pick out a test strip for a blood glucose test, choose between two places for an injection, or wipe off the injection site with a swab.

Puberty and diabetes

Just when you think you have a pretty good handle on helping your child to control blood glucose, along comes puberty. Suddenly you're dealing with unpredictable moods *and* unpredictable blood glucose readings.

Some teenagers may start neglecting diabetes care as part of an overall drive for independence. This can play a role in unexplained high and low blood glucose readings during puberty. In addition, growth- and sex-hormone surges typically cause increased insulin resistance. Your teenager will probably need more insulin during puberty, along with more frequent blood glucose tests to make sure that a mood swing isn't caused by hypoglycemia.

If your teenage daughter has higher blood glucose levels around the time of her period, you and your daughter should talk with her doctor. The doctor may adjust your daughter's treatment regimen to compensate for the influence of the menstrual cycle.

Your teen's self-sufficiency may tempt you to turn diabetes care entirely over to him or her. Don't do it. While it's important for your child to gradually assume more responsibility for diabetes management, parental guidance and support remains crucial to good diabetes control throughout the teen years. But remember that teenagers need to be fully prepared for taking over their diabetes care by the end of high school so they're ready to handle it at college or wherever life takes them.

Ages 4 to 7. Your child may be able to help keep blood glucose records and may enjoy helping to plan meals.

Ages 8 to 11. With supervision and support, your child may be able to perform a finger-stick blood glucose test by age 8 and self-administer insulin by age 10.

Ages 12 to 15. This age group may be ready to self-monitor blood glucose levels under normal circumstances. A child who takes insulin should be able to manage injections or pump infusions with supervision.

> ## Wearing an ID
> No matter what the age, your child needs to wear an identification (ID) tag about diabetes so that others have access to emergency information when needed. Your teen may be more accepting if the ID is a necklace, "dog tag," or bracelet (for the wrist or ankle) that's unique and attractive. Even shoe tags for toddlers are available. You can search the Web for a variety of styles and prices, and many pharmacies also carry them. A wallet card can easily be overlooked and isn't carried all the time, so it may not help during sports activities, for example.

Ages 16 to 18. Your teenager is likely ready to start managing diabetes care independently so that he or she can take over the responsibility by the end of high school. This includes being well prepared to handle possible complications such as hypoglycemia.

Emotional and social issues

Coping with a diagnosis of diabetes is tough for all children and teens. If your child is very young, all the tests and injections may feel like punishment. An older child may be crushed to realize that he or she is different from peers and that diabetes isn't going to go away. Sadness, anger and withdrawal are all normal reactions. However, feelings of hopelessness that last for weeks call for medical attention.

Encourage your child to talk about feelings. Your preschooler may be able to vent emotions by drawing pictures or role-playing with dolls and stuffed animals. Older children (and parents!) may feel better just having a chance to holler, stomp, kick a pillow or cry. Listen to your child without trying to put a positive spin on diabetes. Let your son or daughter know that you're there to help.

Your child may be nervous about telling friends about the diagnosis. Volunteer for practice conversations, and let your child know that whom to tell, when to tell and how much to say is a personal decision.

Your child may want to talk with a trusted teacher or school social worker who can help ease the transition to managing diabetes at school. A local support group for children and teens with diabetes also might make coping easier. Your diabetes educator can put you in touch with resources in your area.

When it's more than sadness

Diabetes increases the risk of depression. Watch for these signs and symptoms in your child:

- Not caring about the things he or she used to
- Having trouble sleeping
- Staying in bed all the time
- Eating a lot more or less than usual
- Losing or gaining a lot of weight without trying
- Difficulty concentrating
- Having anxiety
- Crying a lot
- Expressing a desire to hurt himself or herself or to die

If you think your child may be depressed, seek help right away. Your doctor or diabetes educator can refer your child to a mental health professional.

Diabetes and drinking: A dangerous mix

Your teenager is headed out to a party with friends. Like most parents, you worry about whether alcohol will be served and whether your child will make smart choices if friends are drinking. Have a frank discussion with your teenager about the risks of alcohol.

Alcohol increases the risk of hypoglycemia, and the sugar content of many mixed drinks can raise blood glucose. If your teenager experiences high or low blood glucose while partying with friends, they may think your child is drunk and take no action to help. It's just not worth the risk. Talk to your child about ways to say no if pressured to drink.

Staying healthy by making lifestyle changes

Healthy eating and increased physical activity are key steps to managing diabetes. Your positive attitude and active participation is a crucial part of helping your child make these permanent lifestyle changes.

Tips for healthy eating

There is no diabetes diet. Essentially, it's the same healthy-eating plan that's recommended for everyone, with moderate portions at regular mealtimes. That means eating a variety of fresh fruits and vegetables, whole grains, and fat-free or low-fat dairy products. It also means fewer fried foods, burgers, sodas, pre-packaged muffins and other unhealthy foods. Chances are, everyone in your family needs to make the same improvements to fuel up for a healthy, active life. Over time, children who use insulin need to learn the careful balance between eating habits and insulin needs.

Launch a family project to find tempting, low-fat recipes. Schedule a movie night and set nutritious snacks on the coffee table. Try air-popped popcorn, fat-free or low-fat chips with salsa, veggies with hummus dip, seasoned and baked potato skins, and fruit-and-yogurt parfaits.

These additional tips can help you enlist the whole family in a healthy-eating program:

- Involve your children in helping to prepare meals in age-appropriate ways. They're much more likely to try a new vegetable dish if they helped chop up the ingredients.
- Eat as many family meals together as possible, and keep table conversation to pleasant topics.
- Don't deprive your child or your family of enjoying a dessert, but choose healthier foods. Modify a favorite recipe with the help of your dietitian, try new recipes, and always use appropriate portions. A carefully chosen dessert at the end of a balanced meal is fine every once in a while, and it can help reduce the likelihood that your child will feel deprived.
- Work with your dietitian to include allowances for foods that your family usually enjoys at special celebrations.

Blood sugar vs. blood glucose

You'll likely hear the term *blood sugar* more often than *blood glucose.* The terms mean the same thing. If you decide to use the term blood sugar, make sure that your child understands what it means (explained in Chapter 1).

Eating other types of carbohydrates — not just sugary foods — can make blood sugar (glucose) rise. Even some adults who've had diabetes for many years still think they can't eat any sugar. But they don't realize they're eating too much of other foods that can make their blood glucose rise. The key is moderation. For the full story on healthy eating, see Chapter 4, including "The scoop on sugar," page 60.

Eating away from home

Find out if healthy foods are on the menu in your child's school cafeteria. If they're not, pack a lunch that follows the same nutritious standards you're setting for the family dinner table. Then call the school and encourage better options.

Most children and teenagers also need a couple of snacks during the day. Ward off vending machine temptations by slipping tasty, wholesome options in your child's backpack. Smart choices include:
- Fat-free or low-fat crackers with low-fat cheese
- Whole-grain bread with peanut butter
- A small tortilla topped lightly with low-fat cheese or turkey
- Fresh fruit

If your child is planning a sleepover at a friend's house, call the other parents in advance and — with your child's permission — discuss what food will be served and why you're asking. If they're not planning healthy snacks, tell them you'll send some along with your child, and include enough for the other children to enjoy.

Get active now

Getting active *with* your child is an essential part of making exercise habits stick, and it will improve your health, too. While regular exercise is important, any physical activity has health benefits. Here are just a few easy ideas to get your whole family moving:

- Head out for a walk and explore the sights together.
- Whip the yard into shape: Rake leaves, garden or shovel snow.
- Throw a ball or a Frisbee disc around.
- Go on a bicycling or rollerblading tour of your neighborhood.
- Turn up the radio and have an impromptu dance party.
- If you have young children, get out the chalk and play hopscotch or duck down for a game of hide-and-seek.

Achievement: No limits

If you worry that diabetes might limit the dreams your child can reach for, consider Gary Hall Jr.'s story. Gary had four Olympic swimming medals in his pocket and was training for more when, in 1999, he started noticing that he was always thirsty and his vision was blurred. He was soon diagnosed with type 1 diabetes.

Gary was shocked. There was no history of diabetes in his family, and he had always worked hard to keep in excellent physical condition.

Gary decided he wasn't going to let diabetes stop him. He found a doctor who believed it was possible for him to continue to train and compete. Under his doctor's supervision, Gary dedicated himself to a rigorous schedule of blood glucose testing and treatment and got back in the pool.

At the 2000 Olympic Games in Sydney, Australia, Gary won four more medals. And at the 2004 games in Athens, Greece, he took gold in the 50-meter freestyle and became one of the most decorated Olympic athletes in history.

Diabetes camps

Think your child would savor the chance to hang out with other kids who have diabetes? Look into a diabetes camp provided by the American Diabetes Association. Staff members are trained in diabetes care, and part of their time with campers is focused on sharing tips for good diabetes management. But a lot of time at camp is spent just having fun with friends who'll make your child feel ordinary — in the best possible way. Ask your diabetes educator to help you locate camps near you.

Resist the lure of your TV and computer. Limit children's and teens' time in front of any screen to less than two hours each day, and show them that good health is a family priority by following these same guidelines yourself.

Questions and answers

My baby has diabetes. He can't talk yet and cries for lots of reasons. How can I tell when he has hypoglycemia?
Eventually, you may be able to recognize a particular cry that signals low blood glucose in your baby. Or, you might notice one or more of these signs and symptoms:
- Crankiness
- Pale skin or a bluish tinge on your baby's fingers or lips
- Sweating or trembling
- Clumsiness

If you're in doubt, check your baby's blood glucose level right away. If that's not possible, treat for hypoglycemia anyway. A small amount of fruit juice or glucagon should be enough to bring your baby's blood glucose back up to a healthy level. Your baby's doctor will give you instructions on the right amounts.

My child is at high risk of type 2 diabetes. How often should screening occur?
Check with your child's doctor, but the usual recommendation is to have a fasting blood glucose test every two years, beginning at age 10 or when puberty starts, whichever comes first.

My husband and I miss going out, but we're hesitant to leave our child with a baby sitter. Any suggestions?
Caring for a child with diabetes can strain your emotional and mental health, so make time for enjoyable outside activities. It's likely that trusted relatives and friends would appreciate the chance to help out. Ask if they'd be willing to watch your child on occasion. Or, call people familiar with diabetes and ask for baby sitter recommendations. You might try your diabetes educator, local support groups and other parents of children with diabetes.

Of course, it's also important that you and your child like and trust the sitter. Invite a promising candidate to come by for a visit when there's time to just sit and play with your child for a while. Have the candidate assist with a blood glucose test and give a dose of medicine to your child. If the person seems overwhelmed or treats your child like a patient, move on to the next candidate.

Are teenage girls with diabetes at higher risk of eating disorders?
Yes. According to the American Diabetes Association, teenage girls with type 1 diabetes may be twice as likely as their peers who don't have diabetes to develop eating disorders. This includes gradually starving themselves (anorexia) and forcing themselves to throw up after eating (bulimia).

It may be that having to pay such close attention to food makes girls with diabetes more likely to obsess about their weight. And insulin can be manipulated to cause weight loss.

Eating disorders increase the risk of complications from diabetes. Even in teens without diabetes, eating disorders can be fatal. Signs that your daughter may have an eating disorder include:
- Extreme fluctuations in blood glucose that can't be explained
- Frequent problems with high or low blood glucose
- Not complying with insulin needs
- Obsession with food or with losing weight
- Avoiding being weighed
- Wearing baggy clothes to hide weight loss
- Avoiding meals with the family
- Binge eating
- Excessive exercising
- Irregular menstrual periods or no menstrual periods

If you think your daughter may have an eating disorder, call her doctor. The doctor may arrange for your daughter to see a mental health professional with special training in eating disorders.

Additional resources

Contact these organizations for more information about diabetes, or visit their Web sites. Some groups offer educational materials that are free or that you can buy.

**American Association
of Diabetes Educators**
100 W. Monroe St.
Suite 400
Chicago, IL 60603
(800) 338-3633
E-mail: aade@aadenet.org
www.aadenet.org

American Diabetes Association
Attn: National Call Center
1701 N. Beauregard St.
Alexandria, VA 22311
(800) 342-2383 (800-DIABETES)
E-mail: AskADA@diabetes.org
www.diabetes.org

Canadian Diabetes Association
National Life Building
1400-522 University Ave.
Toronto, ON M5G 2R5, Canada
(800) 226-8464 (800-BANTING)
or (416) 363-0177
E-mail: info@diabetes.ca
www.diabetes.ca

**Centers for Disease Control
and Prevention, Division of
Diabetes Translation**
P.O. Box 8728
Silver Spring MD 20910
(877) 232-3422 toll-free
(877-CDC-DIAB)
E-mail: diabetes@cdc.gov
www.cdc.gov/diabetes

**Diabetes Exercise and
Sports Association**
8001 Montcastle Drive
Nashville, TN 37221
(800) 898-4322
E-mail:
   desa@diabetes-exercise.org
www.diabetes-exercise.org

**International Diabetes
Federation**
Avenue Emile De Mot 19
B-1000 Brussels, Belgium
E-mail: info@idf.org
www.idf.org

Juvenile Diabetes Research Foundation International
120 Wall St.
New York, NY 10005-4001
(800) 533-2873 (800-533-CURE)
E-mail: info@jdrf.org
www.jdrf.org

Mayo Clinic Health Information
www.MayoClinic.com
Search for "diabetes"
    and related terms

National Diabetes Education Program
1 Diabetes Way
Bethesda, MD 20814-9692
(800) 438-5383
E-mail: ndep@info.nih.gov
www.ndep.nih.gov

National Diabetes Information Clearinghouse
1 Information Way
Bethesda, MD 20892-3560
(800) 860-8747
E-mail: ndic@info.niddk.nih.gov
www.diabetes.niddk.nih.gov

National Kidney Education Program
3 Kidney Information Way
Bethesda, MD 20892
(866) 454-3639 toll-free
(866-4-KIDNEY)
E-mail:
    nkdep@info.niddk.nih.gov
www.nkdep.nih.gov

National Kidney Foundation
30 East 33rd St.
New York, NY 10016
(800) 622-9010 or (212) 889-2210
www.kidney.org

Scientific Registry of Transplant Recipients
www.ustransplant.org

United Network for Organ Sharing (UNOS)
P.O. Box 2484
Richmond, VA 23218
(888) 894-6361 toll-free
www.unos.org
www.transplantliving.org

Index

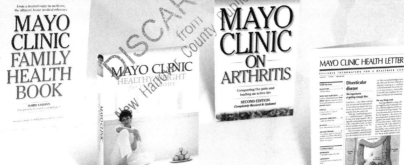

MayoClinic.com Bookstore
Tools for healthier lives

More of the health information you're looking for...

Now the expertise of the world-renowned Mayo Clinic is more accessible to you than ever before.

Mayo doctors and editors produce a wide range of consumer health publications — books and newsletters on topics of interest to millions of health-conscious women and men.

Visit *Bookstore.MayoClinic.com* today and discover our selection of practical, understandable health information...

- *Mayo Clinic Family Health Book,* the ultimate home health reference
- *Mayo Clinic Healthy Weight for EveryBody,* a sensible weight-loss program
- *Mayo Clinic on Arthritis,* one of more than a dozen condition-specific books in our popular "Mayo Clinic on..." series
- *Mayo Clinic Health Letter,* our award-winning newsletter read in more than 750,000 homes every month

These practical, reliable and authoritative publications and many more are available at our online bookstore. Visit today and find more of the health information you're looking for!

Bookstore.MayoClinic.com

Order by calling toll-free (877) 647-6397
Or order online at Bookstore.MayoClinic.com.
Price does not include shipping and handling and applicable sales tax. All prices subject to change.

Mayo Clinic books are available at local bookstores.

DISCARDED from New Hanover County Public Library